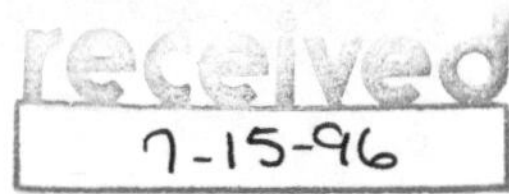

American Medical Association

Physicians dedicated to the health of America

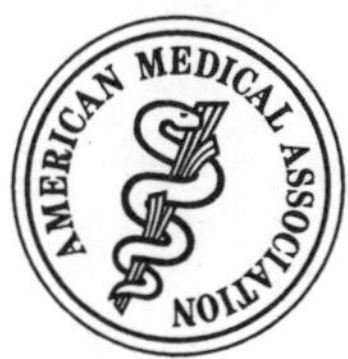

Managing the Medical Practice

The Physician's Handbook for
Successful Practice Administration

Project Manager/Editor: .... Kay Stanley
Project Assistant: .... Joyce Julian
Project Contributor:
Lauretta Mink, CMA, CMM
Art Director: .... Jeff Weir

Published by:

Coker Publishing, LLC —
in affiliation with The Coker Group
3150 Holcomb Bridge Road, Suite 200
Norcross, Georgia 30071
(770) 242-0118

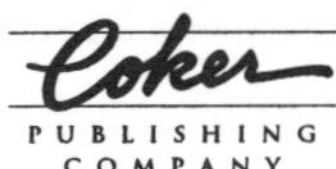

ISBN 0-89970-755-6

©1996 Coker Publishing, LLC

American Medical Association Preface

This book and others contained in the *PRACTICE SUCCESS!*© Series are designed to offer you concrete, practical information on topics that you may sometimes consider the least important aspect of the profession of medicine: the business of running a medical practice. And in some ways, that's how it should be. The long, hard years you dedicated to medical school and residency training were meant to make you an excellent physician, not an excellent businessperson. Caring for patients is and always will be your first priority. But you cannot successfully run a medical practice without planning and without consideration of important business issues. While it takes a minimum of ten years for a person to become a physician, the day a practice opens is the day a physician becomes a small businessperson.

Your many years of superb education probably did not include much information on medical office operations, personnel management, accounting or business law. Yet these business issues are more important than ever before, because the practice of medicine in today's rapidly changing environment is far more complex than ever before. Good business management today is essential to good medical practice. The physician who ignores basic business principles in operating his or her practice may soon face difficulties with suppliers, employees, the government or even patients.

Other pressures today force physicians to search for more efficient ways of running their practices. Most physicians find demands on their time increasing tremendously. There is a daily struggle to build a practice that will earn a steady income, to schedule regular working hours, to deliver quality care to patients and to still have time for relaxation and family.

Developing an efficient practice that runs smoothly makes all of these attainable. The application of good business planning will enable you to spend more time on those things that are most important to you.

This book and the others in the *PRACTICE SUCCESS!*© Series are guides to medical practice management for the new physician and the established physician who wants to survey his or her practice with an eye towards improvement. These books will not provide you with solutions to every challenge that may arise in day-to-day practice. Our goal is to acquaint you with essential business principles and tools, as well as with some new approaches to managing your practice. The knowledge you acquire from this series can be supplemented by information you gather from talking with your colleagues and advisors. You will then be in a position to explore those ideas that promise to achieve the best results for your particular practice situation.

By providing the information in this book and others, the **American Medical Association (AMA)** is not endorsing any one management philosophy or method of delivering health care services. No one approach will meet the objectives of all physicians. Physicians and their staffs will have to decide for themselves what is the best way to manage their individual practices. Finally, this book does not enunciate **AMA** policy. The annual *Policy Compendium* of the **AMA** sets forth our positions on such issues as contracting, medical ethics, managed care and practice management.

We hope that this publication will be useful to you.

The American Medical Association

About The Coker Group

The Coker Group is a national provider of health care consultative and management services assisting physicians, hospitals, and health care systems to better position themselves to be successful in a reformed health care environment. The Coker Group offers the following services for its clients:

Programs and Services:

- Primary Care Physician Network Development

- Practice Valuations and Acquisition Negotiations

- Physician Employment and Compensation Contract Design

- The Facilitation of Group Practice Development

- Physician Practice Management Services

- Management Services Organization (MSO) Development

- Market Share Management Program

- Newly Recruited Physician Services

- Educational Programs

- Evaluation and Consultant Services

- Personnel Productivity Programs

- *PRACTICE SUCCESS!*© and *PRACTICE SUCCESS!*© Series

For more information, contact:

THE
Coker
GROUP

National Consultants to Healthcare Providers

The Coker Group / 3150 Holcomb Bridge Road / Suite 200
Norcross, Georgia 30071 / (770) 242-0118

About The Book

Managing the Medical Practice concerns the complex challenges of medical practice administration. Today's medical practices take diverse organizational shapes and forms. Whether your practice is a large physician group or the business of a solo practitioner, or whether the practice is owned by an outside entity or is a closely held family operation, most management principles similarly apply. The successful operation of a medical practice includes the complex relationship between an employer and an employee; the challenging responsibilities for rendering services and collecting receivables; the complicated duties of running a facility, purchasing supplies and maintaining equipment; the multi-faceted means of managing risk, including understanding various insurance coverages, and a myriad of other aspects of management. All of these responsibilities rest primarily on the shoulders of the practice administrator, who may be assisted in any or all of these by supervisory and specialized personnel at various levels. This book offers sensible systems and guidelines, provided in a direct, forthright manner for the day-to-day management of a medical practice.

Who should read this book?

Anyone interested in the various aspects of medical practice administration will benefit greatly from this book. Whether the reader is the physician, practice administrator, or any member of the staff charged with an area of practice management responsibility, this information will apply to your role. It is a direct guide for all those involved for medical business management, including:

- Owners of medical practices and clinics.
- Managers or supervisors of any medical business.
- Administrators in health care facilities, nursing homes, clinics, and medical practices.

What information can the reader find?

This book covers staff management including personnel law and regulations, leadership, team building, communication and time management skills development. It encompasses financial management including revenue and accounts payable management. It includes operations management with topics such as policies and procedures, facility management, and insurance. And it provides information on the various aspects of risk management, including how to reduce exposure to medical malpractice claims. This work is a "how-to" management tool using simple, straightforward guidelines.

While an attempt is made to review the fundamentals of management, this book is offered with the understanding that the publisher is not engaged in rendering legal, accounting, or other professional services. If legal advice or other expert assistance is required, the services of a competent professional person should be sought.

About the contributors

Lauretta Mink, CMA, CMM, Vice President—Practice Services of The Coker Group, is the principal contributor and author of *Managing the Medical Practice—The Physician's Guide to Successful Practice Administration.* With over 27 years of experience in the health care industry, Ms. Mink works extensively with medical practices in management and personnel training. Her primary areas of expertise include financial management, practice transition, collections, personnel management, and practice development. A talented seminar speaker, she has presented many programs on these topics to physicians and their staffs.

Ms. Mink's prior experience includes serving as Vice President of Operations of a medical management corporation with annual revenues in excess of $15,000,000. Responsibilities included day-to-day supervision of the management of 20 medical practices. Recently, Ms. Mink has been involved with the development and management of an MSO for one of Atlanta's largest hospitals. She is well-prepared to handle the challenges facing physicians today in the rapidly changing health care industry.

Managing the Medical Practice is one of a series of topical books developed for physicians and their staff. Named the *PRACTICE SUCCESS!©* Series, these units are written to provide essential information on medical practice management. This material is compiled and edited by The Coker Group and published by Coker Publishing, LLC. Series contributors, in addition to Ms. Mink, are J. Max Reiboldt, and Kay Stanley, and other members of The Coker Group staff—each of whom bring to the project unique and extensive experience in practice administration and personnel management.

PRACTICE SUCCESS!© is a comprehensive practice management guidebook published by Coker Publishing, LLC, Norcross, GA. This material provides the practice administrator with the essential operational tools and systems to successfully run a medical practice. The complete program consists of a 550+ page manual and includes 77 forms to save time in the daily operation of the practice. Text and forms are available on diskette. A bulletin/update service is also offered.

Managing Editor
Kay B. Stanley

Overview

Managing a medical practice is a complex assignment requiring various skills for handling myriad responsibilities. The successful administration of a medical practice involves the management of personnel, finances, facilities, purchasing and risk. The administrator must be well-acquainted with countless aspects of managed care, and able to make recommendations for participation and compliance. This book offers sensible systems and guidelines, provided in a direct, forthright manner, for the day-to-day management of a medical practice.

The information in this book will help the reader accomplish these objectives:

- Understand the scope and dimension of the administrator's job.

- Develop and enhance skills in leadership, team building, communication and time management.

- Attain knowledge in employee relations including compliance with employment law and occupational law affecting the medical employer.

- Hire only the best; conduct and administer orientation and training, performance appraisals, salary administration, and disciplinary action.

- Increase skill levels in areas of revenue management such as budgeting, purchasing, accounts payable management, and accounts receivable management.

- Implement sound practice policies and procedures for the safety and convenience of the staff and the patients.

- Manage the facilities with efficiency and effectiveness.

- Become knowledgeable of appropriate insurance for the operation of the practice.

- Present the medical practice to the marketplace favorably to increase its market share.

- Manage risk by developing a loss prevention program that includes the physician-patient relationship, proper handling of medical records, and reduction of various exposures to risk.

Practices are organized differently based on the size of the practice, the number of physicians, and the number and authority of various supervisory and technical personnel. All of the information that follows may apply to employees other than the practice administrator. Therefore, the word "administrator" throughout this text means any person within the practice who has responsibility for the function being discussed.

Table of Contents

Chapter 1 – Managing the Staff 1

The Administrator's Role 1

    Administrator's Job Description 2

        Primary Responsibilities 2

        Specific Duties of the Job 2

        Job Qualifications and Requirements 4

        Job Relationships 4

        Authority Boundaries 4

        Interviewing Practice Administrator Candidates 4

Leadership 5

    Five Keys to Successful Leadership 6

Team Building 7

    Benefits of Teamwork 7

    Managing Conflict 7

    Motivating Employees 8

Effective Communication 9

    Staff Meetings 9

    Active Listening 10

Time Management 12

    Seven Key Activities 13

    Personal Time Management 13

    Employee Time Management 15

    Physician Time Management 15

    Summary Report 16

Chapter 2 – Employee Relations 17

Statutes Overview 17

    Fair Labor Standards Act of 1938 (FLSA) 17

    Equal Pay Act of 1963 19

    The Civil Rights Act of 1964, Title VII 19

    Age Discrimination in Employment Act of 1967 (ADEA) 19

    Equal Employment Opportunity Act of 1972 19

    Pregnancy Discrimination of 1978 19

Consolidated Omnibus Budget Reconciliation Act of 1985 (COBRA)......................................19

Americans with Disabilities Act of 1990 (ADA)..19

Family Medical Leave Act of 1963...20

Occupational Laws...20

Workers' Compensation Law 20

Dual Capacity Doctrine 22

Establishing a Safety Policy 22

Handling an Accident..22

First Report of Injury Report...22

OSHA Work Place Requirements 23

Labor Laws 23

Consolidated Omnibus Budget Reconciliation Act of 1985 (COBRA)......................................23

Sexual Harassment...24

Definition of Sexual Harassment 24

Responsibilities...24

Preventive Actions 24

Americans with Disabilities Act (ADA)..25

Anti-Discrimination Provisions 25

Reasonable Accommodation 25

Enforcement 26

Age Discrimination in Employment Act (ADEA) 26

Enforcement 26

Federal Recordkeeping Requirements 27

List for Retention 27

Posting Requirements 29

Employment Categories 30

Executive 30

Administrative 30

Professional...30

At-Will Contracts 31

Chapter 3 – Personnel Management...33

Hiring Only the Best 33

Recruitment Process...33

Developing a Recruitment Process 33

Preparing the Job Description..33

Using Job Descriptions..34

Creating a Candidate Profile 34

Place the Advertisement 35

Review the Resumés 35
Telephone Screening of Candidates 36
Setting Appointments for Interviews 36
Interviewing 37
Checking References 39
Making the Offer 39
Setting Up the Personnel File...40
The Probationary Period..40
Credentialing of Health Care Providers 41
Hiring Independent Contractors 42

Outsourcing/Employee Leasing...42

Sample Job Offer Letter...43

Orientation and Training 44
Training for the New Position...44
Final Training Tips 45

Performance Appraisals and Salary Administration 45
Preparing for the Performance Appraisal 46
Twenty-Two Tips for Productive Performance Discussions....................................47
Salary Administration..50

Disciplinary Action..51
Performance Problems...51
Misconduct..51
Termination...52

The Employee Handbook 53

Chapter 4 – Financial Management...57

The Operating Budget 57
Benchmarking 57
Personnel Costs 59
Staffing Ratios by Specialty 59
Major Expenses by Specialty 60
Medical and Administrative Expenses...61
Purchasing 61
Outsourcing...61
Vendor Relations...62
Inventory Control 62
Ordering Logs 63
Bartering 63

Occupancy Expense 63

Malpractice Insurance 64

Legal and Accounting Fees 64

Service Contracts 64

Petty Cash 64

Petty Cash Fund 64

Tracking Revenues 65

Determining Profitability 65

Revenue and Expense 65

Patient Cost Analysis 66

Accounts Payable Management 66

Definition 66

Purchasing 66

Paying Bills 67

Payroll 67

Accounts Receivable Management 68

Definition 68

Patient Policy Education 68

Collecting at the Time of Service 68

The Written Financial Payment Policy 69

Patient Billing 69

The Written Collection Policy 69

Purpose of a Written Collection Policy 69

Keys to Successful Collecting 70

Collections 70

Collection Ratio 70

Terminating the Physician-Patient Relationship 70

Fees 71

Fee Analysis 71

Cost Procedure Analysis 72

Chapter 5 – Operations Management 73

Practice Policies and Procedures 73

Procedure Manual 73

Appointment Scheduling and Registration Policy 74

Appointments 74

Reception and Registration 76

Facility Management 76
    Office Environment..76
        Suggestions for Pleasant Reception Area 77
    Facility Management 77
    The Physical Plant 77
Interior Office Checklist 79
Facility Evaluation 80

Chapter 6 – Managed Care 81

Practice Enhancement 81
    Patient Satisfaction Survey...81
    Patient Services and Amenities 84
    Marketing in a Managed Care Market 86
        Ten Ways to Show Health Plans How Good You Are 86
        Strategies for Managed Care Marketplace 87
        Health Plan Profile..87
        Tracking Pre-Certification 87

Telephone Triage Guidelines 88

Chapter 7 – Risk Management in the Medical Office 91

    Developing a Loss Prevention Program..91
    Scheduling...91
    Billing and Collections 92
    Environment..93
    Medical Equipment 93
    Emergencies 93
    Confidentiality 94
    Handling Patient Complaints 94
    Termination of the Patient/Physician Relationship 94
    Rights of the Patient..95
    Consent to Treatment..95
    Informed Consent to Treatment 96
    Patient's Obligations 96
    Physician's Obligations 96
    The Medical Record 97
    Authorization to Release Records 97
    Key Elements of a Good Medical Record 97

Exhibits...99

Monthly Statistics Form (Exhibit 1) 101
Employee Safety Orientation Checklist (Exhibit 2-1) 102
Accident/Injury Report — Employer (Exhibit 2-2) 103
Accident/Injury Report — Employee (Exhibit 2-3) 104
Accident/Injury Report — Witness (Exhibit 2-4) 105
Exposure Incident Protocol (Exhibit 2-5)..106
Exposure Incident Report (Exhibit 2-6) 107
Post Exposure Incident Form — Source (Exhibit 2-7)...............................109
Post Exposure Incident Form — Exposed (Exhibit 2-8) 110
Sample Job Descriptions (Exhibits 3-1, 3-2, 3-3) 111
Employee Performance Appraisal Form (Exhibit 3-4) 115
Salary Change Recommendation (Exhibit 3-5) 119
Corrective Action Form (Exhibit 3-6) 120
Terminating Employee Checklist (Exhibit 3-7) 122
Practice Management Statistics (Exhibit 4-1) 123
Major Expenses by Specialty (Exhibit 4-2) 124
Petty Cash Fund (Exhibit 4-3) 125
Summary Report for Tracking Practice Growth and Profitability (Exhibit 4-4) 126
Patient Information Registration Form (Exhibit 5-1)................................127
Guide to Estimated Times for Common Medical Office Procedures (Exhibit 5-2) 128
Appointment Schedule (Exhibit 5-3)...129
Patient Satisfaction Survey (Exhibit 6-1) 130
Health Plan Profile (Exhibit 6-2) 132
Incident Report Form (Exhibit 7-1)...133
Patient Complaint Log (Exhibit 7-2) 134
Sample Discharge Letter (Exhibit 7-3) 135
Authorization for Release of Medical Records (Exhibit 7-4)...................136
Medical Records Checklist Form (Exhibit 7-5) 137
Medication Record Form (Exhibit 7-6) 138

Bibliography/Resources...139

Index...141

Managing the Staff

Because the administrative role in a medical practice varies with the size of the practice, the number of physicians, and the number and authority of various supervisory and technical personnel, all of the information that follows may apply to employees other than the practice administrator. Therefore, the word "administrator" is used throughout this text to mean any person within the practice who has responsibility for the function being discussed.

The Administrator's Role

The role of the practice administrator is similar to that of the vice president of a corporation. The president (in this case, the physician) makes the decisions and sets the guidelines and delegates to the vice president (the practice administrator), who implements them. The administrator must possess the ability and the understanding of three basic elements that make up a successful business operation:

- **Revenue Management**
  The primary responsibility of the practice administrator is to maintain good collections. The success of the medical practice is founded on the premise that no matter what the financial statements might indicate as profit, the ability to maintain adequate cash flow is of primary importance.

- **Business Administration**
  In the well-run practice, the practice administrator has the support of the physician and the staff members. The practice administrator develops a knowledge of employment law, maintains good employee relations and supervises employees with understanding and openness.

- **Effective Communication**
  Effective communication is vital to realizing the goals for a successful practice. The practice administrator must be a skillful, two-way communicator, able to listen, ask the right questions, and convey essential information to the physician and to the staff. Employees must be heard when there are suggestions and concerns.

- **Employee Organization**
  A key function of managing is delegation. Managing does not mean doing the work of others. The successful practice administrator delegates tasks and supervises their completion.

All administrative employees report to the practice administrator. While clinical employees may report directly to the physician on clinical matters, in administrative issues such as vacations, employee relations, work hours, etc., they abide by the decisions of the practice administrator.

This role is communicated to the staff by the physician. In larger practices, other employees may serve in administrative or supervisory capacities as well, or even be part of the larger structure of a practice management company with a complex organization chart.

The physician should be very careful not to make a personnel or management decision when an employee attempts to circumvent the practice administrator on an administrative issue. For example, if the physician gives an employee permission for a day off when that request has already been denied by the office administrator, it severely undermines the practice administrator's authority.

When an employee approaches the physician on an administrative issue, he should state, "I understand your concern or your need, but you will have to check with the practice administrator for that answer. Because he knows all the specifics surrounding your eligibility, the decision can be made according to practice policy."

A successful practice is one in which the physician and administrator work closely to support each other's efforts.

The Administrator's Job Description

Reports To:

Physician in charge of Personnel

Primary Responsibilities:

- Manages the daily operation of the medical practice including administrative, financial, personnel, clerical, housekeeping, maintenance, and purchasing functions.
- Plans, programs, allocates, and assigns duties to the employees. Monitors activities and operations to ensure that the practice successfully meets its objectives.

Specific Duties of the Job:

- Supervises and coordinates the activities of all practice personnel.
- Organizes and assigns duties to employees related to bookkeeping, payroll, collections, insurance, secretarial support, medical records, telephone procedures, housekeeping, appointment scheduling, patient flow, patient relations and coordination (with physician and professional staff) of clinical activities.
- Monitors the duties assigned to practice personnel to ensure that employees are performing their assignments in a manner designed to maintain a high level of patient care and job efficiency.
- Maintains efficient flow of work throughout the practice by evaluating procedures.
- Standardizes procedures and initiates changes where necessary. Constantly reviews procedures to strive for more efficient ways to conduct business and improve patient relations.

- Directs operations to prepare and retain records, files, reports and correspondence according to various governmental and practice standards. Prepares and implements a records retention and disposition program for the practice.

- Helps establish, revise and implement practice policy and operating procedures.

- Interviews, tests, hires, counsels, and terminates employees and verifies information on employment applications. Arranges for background checks on applicants for employment. Conducts periodic performance and salary reviews.

- Prepares, maintains, and provides security for personnel records. Retains applications from applicants for employment.

- Reviews and approves weekly time records of all practice employees. Approves all sick and emergency leave according to practice policy. Establishes and schedules vacations for all employees (including coordination of physician's vacations, education leaves, etc.).

- Develops and administers an on-the-job training program for new and current employees as required.

- Schedules and conducts periodic office staff meetings to inform the staff of changes in the practice's policy, to update and educate staff, and to resolve and prevent problems. Prepares and retains minutes of all meetings.

- Schedules meetings for (and with) the physician. Notifies those who are to attend. Coordinates the logistics of the meetings. Attends physician's meetings when appropriate. Reports on the status of practice operation, equipment and financial operations. Takes (or arranges for) minutes and maintains records of each meeting. Prepares agenda for all meetings.

- Maintains the physician's master schedule and coordinates activities.

- Helps to maintain and coordinate care of the physical plant and equipment. Ensures routine maintenance of equipment (in coordination with professional staff). Ensures cleanliness, organization, functional operating condition, and appropriate decor.

- Prepares and distributes payroll and keeps appropriate records.

- Manages all financial and organization books maintained by the practice.

- Prepares or helps to prepare other financial and statistical reports on a scheduled basis and as requested by the physician.

- Works with the practice's accountant, attorney, and other support agencies as required.

- Reviews the accounting system to ensure it is operating within the limits of well defined internal control standards.

- Works with the physician and accountant to prepare a budget for the practice. Annually compares actual and projected budget and helps to make appropriate adjustments to ensure adherence to the budget.

- Reviews all invoices and statements from vendors for payment. Ensures receipt of all items billed. Checks for appropriate discounts, etc. Coordinates with physician in ordering supplies, purchasing equipment or making other capital expenditures. Secures competitive bids for supplies and equipment when appropriate.

- Monitors outstanding accounts receivable. Works with office staff, credit and insurance clerks, etc., to ensure constant monitoring of the balances outstanding.

- Initiates steps to reduce the accounts receivable.

- Performs other duties as directed by physician to achieve desired results.

Job Qualifications and Requirements:

- Has high school diploma. Completion of an accredited practice administration program. Bachelor of Science degree preferred. Adequate experience may be substituted (in whole or in part) for educational requirements at the discretion of the physician.

- Has employment history indicating progressive, responsible experience in a hospital, business office, or medical practice.

- Is self-motivated, honest, energetic, and committed.

- Possesses the tact and interpersonal skills necessary to deal effectively with patients, physicians, employees, and others. Has ability to motivate the employees within the environment of the practice.

- Possesses the ability to think clearly and to make judgmental decisions in initiating business and office policy.

- Possesses a knowledge of modern office equipment, including computer systems and procedures to allow smooth and efficient operation of the practice. Has ability to operate and instruct others in the use of common office machines and willingness to learn new machines and procedures.

- Possesses the ability to advise the physician in areas of practice and business management, to maximize patient care and service, and to direct efficient and profitable operations of the practice. Serves as the liaison between other outside services and consultants (attorneys, CPAs, insurance agents, etc.) and the practice.

- Agrees to be legally bonded.

- Agrees to a careful background check.

Job Relationships:

- Directly supervises all non-clinical personnel. Indirectly manages (through the head nurse) all clinical personnel.

- Works with and receives supervision from the physician.

Authority Boundaries:

- All major policy and operating decisions are carried out by the practice administrator but are made by the physician.

Interviewing Practice Administrator Candidates

The practice administrator acts as the physician's agent in employee supervision, collection of fees and the control of practice expenses. Careful selection of an experienced, intelligent person for this role is of vital importance.

Following is a list of questions the physician should ask potential candidates for the position of practice administrator. If the candidate is unable to give positive, thorough answers to these questions, the physician may choose to look further for a more qualified applicant.

- Why did you (or do you plan to) leave your last job as office manager/administrator?

- What was the one thing you liked most about that job?

- If you could change anything about your last job, what would it be?
  What else would you change?

- Tell me how you handled payments on account?
  - Who opened the mail?
  - Who tallied checks received?
  - Who posted payments to patient's account receivable?
  - Who made bank deposits?

- What was average percentage of accounts receivable over 90 days old?

- What collection procedures did you use?

- Were practice profits increasing or decreasing?

- What kind of patient procedures did the doctor perform in the office?

- Have you ever had an outside firm review your fee schedule and coding?

- Are you a member of any professional association?

- What trade journals or magazines do you read?

- Where did you buy practice supplies?

- How did you decide where to buy?

- What do you handle patient copay? (When and how is money collected?)

- How much did you discount fees (%)?

- How many claims filed were denied? How did you handle denied claims?

- Who determined what hospital to use when admitting a patient?

- How did you select another physician to refer patients?

- Did you receive referrals from other practices? How did you notify referring physician?

- How many managed care contracts did the practice participate in? What was the term and
  how were they renewed?

Leadership

Leadership is the most studied and least understood of all the social sciences. Leadership is
often confused with management; however, leadership and management are profoundly
different. Both are important.

To *manage* means "to bring about; to accomplish; to have charge of or responsibility for; to
conduct." *To lead* is "to influence; to guide in direction, course, action, opinion." Managers are
people who do things right; leaders do the right thing. To summarize, management produces
efficiency and leadership produces effectiveness.

The successful practice is both managed and led by various members of the staff. To be a
successful leader you must first establish your personal, professional and practice goals. Your

practice's goals and the way you communicate them to the employees enables you to effectively manage and control your daily responsibilities.

The medical practice will not survive health care reform without efficient management, and the efficient practice will not be successful without effective leadership. Practices must be led to adapt to changing conditions.

Personnel management is at the heart of leadership. People like and follow others not for who they are or what they know, but for how they make them feel.

Teaching is a leadership responsibility. Help your staff have pride and satisfaction in their work. Let them know that their individual contributions are needed and respected.

Five Keys to Successful Leadership

1. **Always accept people as they are, not what you would like them to be.**
    Begin with each employee's basic skills and personality. Take the time to discover what their goals are. If they have no goals, encourage them to set some. Help them to see their individual value to the practice. Give them every opportunity to build on any skill they have or any they wish to attain.

2. **Approach a relationship in terms of the present, not the past.**
    If an employee needs discipline or correction, take care of it as soon as possible. Make the proper notes in their file and then forget about it. Do not always think of that person as a troublemaker. Wipe the slate clean.

3. **Treat your employees with the same courteous attention that you extend to patients and personal acquaintances.** The leader can set the work tone for others. Thank them each day for being there and doing their job. Employees do not continue in a position simply because they are well paid. Spoken appreciation, a sense of belonging, and the acknowledgement that they are making an important contribution to the practice are far more important to most employees than money.

4. **Trust others, even if the risk seems great.**
    Delegation, a vital part of effective leadership, requires a measure of trust. Trust your employees with important tasks. They will probably surprise you with their abilities and performance!

5. **Develop the ability to do without constant approval and recognition.**
    A successful leader understands the responsibilities of the people he leads. Acquaint yourself with each employee's role and the functions necessary to perform the tasks. When possible, spend time actually doing the employee's job.   Be willing to invest time and effort in learning the requirements of the work necessary to run the practice. A leader understands and leads effectively.

Empowering a work force requires knowledge, attentiveness, creativity, and acceptance of risk. In a word, it takes **LEADERSHIP.**

Team Building

The traditional definition of a team is a group of people who share responsibility for the decisions that affect them all. Teamwork means contribution and collaboration. It requires both the freedom and the ability to participate fully.

Building a successful medical staff team requires listening, asking for ideas, and communicating the practice's goals to the employees.

Benefits of Teamwork

- A smoothly functioning team better serves the patient.

- Members of a smoothly functioning team experience greater job satisfaction.

- A smoothly functioning team reduces the risk of malpractice.

Teamwork is most likely achieved through impartial management. Factions may tend to develop between clinical and front office personnel and invisible lines be drawn. Guard against this tendency. Instead, encourage the physicians and clinical personnel to interact more with the front office staff. Sometimes, saying "thank you" at the end of the day is all that is required.

Cross-training encourages teamwork. Medical assistants should be trained to answer the telephones, use the computer, check in a patient, make an appointment and file charts. Administrative employees should be capable of taking vital signs, chaperoning a patient to an exam room, scheduling a lab test or surgery, and preparing an exam room for the next patient.

By working closely together to understand each other's needs, both the clinical and administrative staff will develop an appreciation for the problems that exist on both sides of that "invisible line." For a fully functioning team to operate smoothly, employees must understand their own roles and how their roles interact with and affect others. Cross-training encourages this understanding.

Note to Physician: You are encouraged to work with and support your administrator. She has the well-being of your practice in mind. Back her administrative decisions. Meet with the administrator on a regular basis to remain well-informed of practice matters.

Managing Conflict

Conflict occurs. Managing the conflict requires a great deal of patience, understanding and finesse. Conflict should not be suppressed, nor should it be allowed to escalate to open clashes. In effective teams, disagreement is perceived as healthy and is handled by promoting open discussion on the topic. The administrator's role is to make the team responsible for solving problems. As soon as the administrator says, "I'll take care of it," other parties feel absolved from the responsibility of resolving the conflict.

Most conflict between employees arises out of personality differences. One of the most positive, long-lasting and informative solutions to personality conflicts is to have all employees take personality/psychological tests. When test results are presented to the staff, have each employee discuss his/her approach to the job in light of the test findings. Discuss how they could better relate to employees of a different type.

Another common source of conflict in an organization results from what we will call the *"Equity Theory."* According to the *Equity Theory*, whether the employee is really being treated fairly is not relevant. Each person responds to his surroundings based on his subconscious judgment of equality.

It works like this:

> *Mary is on time every day, is prepared to go to work immediately and gives 110 percent all day long. Loretta is often tardy and slow to get started, but does an adequate job all day.*
>
> *If Mary perceives that Loretta receives the same pay and benefits and gets the same praise and encouragement from management, Mary will begin to feel an inequity and build resentment. Eventually she will modify her work habits to match Loretta's. She will justify this by saying to herself, "Why should I work this hard when Loretta does half the work I do and receives the same rewards?"*
>
> *There are many opportunities to modify behaviors. Simply telling Mary that she is doing a wonderful job may be all that is required. Other options may include a small raise or bonus for Mary, or an adjustment of responsibilities.*

Being aware of the *Equity Theory* allows the practice administrator to analyze the office environment from yet another angle. There are many opportunities to modify Mary's perception.

The *Equity Theory* applies to everyone. The entire staff, including the practice administrator and the doctors, is sensitive to being treated fairly. It is amazing how a kind word from the administrator can increase a person's sense of job satisfaction.

Motivating Employees — What Do They Really Want?

Recognizing why a person is working provides clues for encouraging the employee to work more effectively. Most people work for a number of reasons. The two most basic are money and experience.

According to Abraham Maslow's, *Hierarchy of Needs*, every person has five levels of needs. Each person will sacrifice a higher level of need to satisfy a lower level.

- Level One: Physiological: the most basic need — air, water, sleep, food.
- Level Two: Security — residence, money, job.
- Level Three: Social — friendship, acceptance, love.
- Level Four: Ego — respect, esteem, status.
- Level Five: Self-actualization — creativity, serving mankind, self-fulfillment.

The administrator can encourage and assist employees in reaching a higher level of need. It will require an investment of time. Informally meet with each employee to review and clarify their personal and professional goals. They may not refer to them as goals, but as a "want list." They are goals just the same. The challenge is to align the employee's goals and needs with the goals and needs of the organization.

What can you offer to help the employee reach a goal? Does your receptionist want to become an administrator? If so, allow her to assist you in functions that will broaden her experience and knowledge. At the same time, you are preparing someone to cover for you in a pinch. For this approach to be effective, the employee must believe that improved performance will help her reach her goal.

"Thank you" bonuses can be an employee motivator. It is not the amount of money, but the thought behind it that rewards the employee who has expended extra effort. Other expressions of appreciation are remembrances on Secretary's Day, birthdays, etc.

Effective Communication

Staff Meetings

Staff meetings require time. While you are in the lounge chatting, work is not being done, and worst of all, the telephone is not being answered. So why stop office activity to sit and talk? **Because it Pays!** Effective communication benefits practice operation.

- Staff meetings save time by:
  - Reducing interruptions during the work day to answer questions.
  - Eliminating task repetitions because someone did not know about a recent change.
  - Lessening the interchange necessary to make a decision.

- Staff meetings increase productivity by:
  - Clarifying *who* is going to do *what* duties *when*.
  - Answering specific questions staff members have about their duties.
  - Reducing incidences of "crisis" management

- Staff meetings generate better decisions by:
  - Deriving input from staff members who provide different views.
  - Setting aside a structured time for making decisions through analysis and contemplation.

Regular staff meetings are the best vehicles for effective communication. Encourage the team to share ideas for improvement, cost containment and patient relations. During these meetings, the physician or practice administrator should share details about the practice, talk about the changing health care environment, and explore ideas about how the practice should prepare for these transformations.

Discuss changes in CLIA, OSHA and Medicare guidelines at these meetings. Even if the administrative staff is not directly affected by the government programs, they should still be knowledgeable of the guidelines and how they affect the practice.

Here are some tips for an effective staff meeting:

- Have an agenda and stick to it.
- Limit meetings to one hour.
- Encourage the physicians to attend.
- Make meetings mandatory.
- Encourage everyone to speak.

- Avoid using staff meetings for disciplinary actions or reprimands.

- Keep the meetings positive and "upbeat." (No gripe sessions allowed.)

- Meet each week; biweekly meetings are acceptable.

- Let each employee be responsible for planning at least one meeting a year. The employee in charge should request input from the rest of the staff to plan the agenda.

- Have at least two meetings a year about "fun" issues. An example of an upbeat meeting is to have everyone share something positive that is going on in her personal life. This is a good time for each employee to explore a personal or professional goal and solicit everyone's support and help. The physicians should attend these meetings, too, to learn more about their staff.

During staff meetings, the practice administrator should explain the costs involved in the operation of the practice. Most staff members see only the revenue side of the business and have no perception of how much revenue is spent on overhead. Efficient office procedures control overhead. Therefore, it is important to seek ideas on cost containment and reduction from employees.

Staff meetings provide an ideal time to discuss ways to improve patient relations. Patient relations can be focused on the *Golden Rule: "Do unto others as you would have them do unto you."* In other words, treat patients the way you want to be treated when you are the patient.

Active Listening

Unlike hearing, listening does not happen automatically; it is an intellectual and emotional process. Usually a listener's feelings, composed of prior knowledge and experiences with the speaker, interfere with the intellectual portion of listening that analyzes and understands what is being said.

Effective listening is hard work. The average listener understands and retains only about 50 percent of a conversation. The percentage drops to 25 percent within 48 hours. As a consequence of poor listening, there is a misconception of what is being said. This results in the poor listener offering the speaker faulty or inappropriate advice on resolving a perceived problem. The poor listener may even address a totally different problem from one communicated. Often, such communication leaves the speaker feeling that the listener either does not care or does not know anything about the problem.

Following are typical complaints from employees about an administrator's listening skills:

- He does all the talking; I go in with a problem and never get a chance to open my mouth.

- She interrupts me when I talk.

- He never looks at me when I talk. I'm not sure he's listening.

- She makes me feel as though I'm wasting her time.

- Her facial expressions and body language keep me guessing about whether she is listening to me.

- He stays on the surface of the conversation or problem.

There are four categories of listeners:

Non-Listener

Fakes attention while thinking about unrelated matters. Too busy preparing response to
listen to what is being said. Rarely interested in what anyone else has to say. Must
always have the last word.

Marginal Listener

Hears the sounds and words but does not really listen. Superficial listener. Stays on the
surface of the problem; never risks searching deeper. Postpones problems into the future.
Easily distracted by own thinking and environment. The marginal listener frequently gives the
speaker the impression that she is being listened to and understood. The speaker goes away
thinking that everything is resolved, only to be even more devastated when the problem
continues because the listener failed to take action.

Valuative Listener

Actively tries to hear what the speaker is saying but is not making an effort to understand the
speaker's intent. More concerned with content than feelings of the speaker. Remains
emotionally detached. Disregards the speaker's vocal intonation, body language, and
facial expressions. Typically great in semantics, facts, and statistics while poor in
sensitivity, empathy, and understanding.

Active Listener

Attempts to see things from the speaker's point of view. Listens for the content, intent, and
feeling of the message. Non-verbally communicates to the speaker that he is truly listening
and is interested in hearing what the speaker wants to say. Tries to get a deeper
understanding of the other person. Listens not only to what is said and how it is said, but
also to what is not being said. Uses questions to encourage speaker to extend the
conversation and clarify the message. Probes areas that need to be developed further in order
to get a better picture of what the speaker is trying to communicate.

Here are stimulators that will help you become an *active listener*:

- It is impossible to listen and talk at the same time. The only interruption a speaker likes
  is applause.

- Listen for the speaker's main ideas. Ask yourself: What is the speaker's message?

- Fight off distractions. Resist the tendency to listen for quirks in delivery.

- Try not to get angry. Emotions of any kind hinder the listening process.

- Do not trust important data to memory. Take brief notes.

- Let others tell their story first. You will then have more information on which to base
  your response.

- Empathize with the speaker. Make an effort to see the speaker's point of view.

- Paraphrase the speaker's ideas and concepts and repeat them back to him in order to
  demonstrate understanding.

The traits of an *active listener* can be summarized with three easy-to-remember actions: *Sensing, Attending,* and *Responding.*

- *Sensing* is the ability to recognize and appreciate the silent messages that the speaker is sending.

- *Attending* is the verbal, vocal, and visual messages that the active listener sends to the speaker indicating attentiveness, receptiveness, and acknowledgement of the speaker.

- *Responding* occurs when the listener stimulates the speaker to provide more details, makes the speaker feel understood, and encourages the speaker to reflect upon the problem or concern to develop a better understanding of the situation.

There is power in listening. When you listen to others, genuinely listen. They will tell you how best to approach them in meeting their needs. People work hardest at meeting their own needs. Therefore, structure their duties so they may satisfy their personal and professional goals by accomplishing the goals of the practice. In an efficient practice, the needs of the staff and the needs of the practice will be aligned.

Time Management

The first step to effective time management is to realize that we can never effectively manage "time." We can only effectively manage ourselves.

Many practice administrators use some type of "time management" techniques advertised or recommended by a friend or coworker. Unfortunately, none of these completely resolve time management problems. Only two things are important for learning about time management.

- ***Realizing you can't do it all***

- ***Organizing and executing around priorities***

We tend to believe we have accomplished something or had a productive day if we can check off several things on our "to do" list. Yet, we may not have accomplished one thing that improves the three critical areas of the practice:

- Patient care

- Revenue enhancement

- Cost containment

Most of us suffer from an *urgency addiction.* There is a good chance that urgency is your fundamental operational pattern. Some of us are so used to the adrenaline rush of handling crises that we are dependent on it for energy and a sense of worth and accomplishment. While it may be stressful, it makes us feel validated and useful.

For some, the mind-set may be, "Whenever there is trouble, we ride into town with our six-shooter, gun the varmint down and valiantly ride off into the sunset." Our instant results bring instant gratification. Everywhere we turn, *urgency addiction* is reinforced in our lives and in our culture.

To be effective time administrators, we must concentrate on what is important instead of what is urgent. Learning to concentrate on the *important* reduces our crisis mode and our *urgency addiction*. The "important" eventually becomes the "urgent." The strategy is to act on the "important" before it becomes the "urgent."

Important things fall under seven key activities:

- Improving communications with people

- Better preparation

- Better planning and organization

- Taking better care of yourself

- Seizing new opportunities

- Personal development

- Empowerment

Rule #1: Delegate

Many practice administrators (usually because of a misplaced sense of responsibility) want to control everything. This unrealistic outlook brings trouble in the long run. If this is your tendancy, your star may burn brightly for a few months or even years, but you will eventually "burn out" and things will not get done.

Delegation is *the most effective* time management tool. ***Do not be afraid to delegate responsibility to others for fear that it threatens your job.*** If the employees you manage do a good job, it reflects well on you. The true responsibility of a leader is to teach others and allow them to learn new skills. As a manager, it is very rewarding to watch someone you have trained and encouraged improve their skills and level of efficiency.

The rules of successful delegation are simple:

- Give specific instructions for the job to be done — written is best.

- Monitor their progress without "checking up on them."

- Set definite time lines for accomplishments and completion of tasks.

- Give encouragement consistently.

Rule #2: Organize and Prioritize

Personal Time Management

Look at your own schedule and assure yourself you are working on the *important* things — not just the *urgent* ones. Take a note pad and begin listing all the things you want to do when you "get around to it." Include your professional and personal goals. Add to the list as you think of things.

- Planning requires more than writing a daily "to do" list. First, a "to do" list limits vision. Daily planning often misses important things that can only be seen from a broader perspective. Looking at your work and personal life over the next year and five years will allow you to continually work on the important things and keep you out of the crisis management trap. Plan every month at least 30 days in advance; 90 days is better. Start your plan by writing down your continuing functions. Enter on your calendar on the day of the month periodic activities such as sending out statements, paying bills, making payroll, conducting performance appraisals and making collection calls.

- Look at your list of "around to its" and plan on doing at least one each month. Plan for it. Be selfish. Be protective, not allowing others to interrupt or control your time. Take responsibility for what you accomplish.

- Next, set up your coming week. Prioritize what is important.

- Finally, make your "to do" list for the coming day.

- Write everything down. Carry a small notebook with you everywhere. Make notes or reminders to yourself as you remember things so nothing is forgotten. Write down your ideas and thoughts.

- Batch your work. Increase your productivity by setting aside specific times for certain tasks, such as returning calls, reviewing the mail, etc. Keep all the information or paperwork for each project in a pocket folder. Work on one project at a time in the order of its priority. Allow one or two hours for working on each project; then go on to the next one.

- Carry a portable tape recorder with you in your car. If you have a long commute, use the time in the car for thinking and planning. When an idea or thought comes to you, record it on your tape recorder.

- Use your voice mail as a reminder tool. Record a message to yourself about important meetings or deadlines.

- Allow time for reading and education. Be informed about the changing health care industry. Read all your managed care contracts. Learn about capitation and how to calculate capitation rates. Read about various integration models and the changes in reimbursement patterns.

- Always strive to improve your own skills and increase your talents.

- Avoid taking work home. If you need to play catch-up, come in early or stay late. Personal time is for home and family. It will not benefit you or the practice if you use personal time for work.

- If you are serious about your job, be first in the morning and last out in the evening.

- Set goals. Write them down on 3" x 5" cards and put them in a prominent place such as on your mirror, on your desk, or in your car. If you believe you can do something, you can. Keep a positive attitude about reaching your goals.

- Strive for patience.

- As you begin each day, focus on your two or three primary goals.

- Set a time limit on activities. Use a timer.

- Let your staff know when you do not wish to be disturbed and when you have an "open door."

- Use the **TRAF** method for handling the mail. Look at each piece of mail and decide immediately if you will:

  - **Toss** it in the trash.

  - **Refer** or delegate it to someone else along with the proper instructions.

  - **Act** on it yourself. Do it immediately if you can complete it in ten minutes or less.

  - **File** it immediately in your own files, or put it in a desk top tray marked "to be filed." Assign filing responsibilities to a staff member. Filing should be done daily.

- Ask yourself, "What is the best use of my time right now?"

Employee Time Management

- Have a "stand up" meeting every morning for ten minutes. Include the physician if possible.

  - Review the schedule for any special orders or circumstance.

  - Give instructions to the staff for jobs that need to be done.

  - Discuss with the physician any calls he may have received at home.

  - Get information from the physician that is required for accurate billing of services, diagnoses or procedures done in the emergency room, hospital or nursing home.

- Develop a *Practice Policies and Procedures Manual* that defines every job function. Have each employee contribute to the manual by providing an outline of his/her tasks/functions and how they are handled. Written policies and procedures are a great time saver, excellent orientation and training resource, and a fundamental part of risk management. (Also see Chapter 5, page 73, *Practice Policies and Procedure Manual.*)

- Encourage your employees to use a daily "to do" list. Help them develop daily and weekly goals. Use the annual performance appraisal for helping employees set personal and professional goals for the coming year. Do not allow them to set goals and then forget about them. Rather, interface with them about their goals throughout the year. Offer encouragement and praise profusely; offer help only on request.

Physician Time Management

The administrator can assist the physician in managing his time more efficiently. The following are a few suggested time management techniques.

- **Scheduling patients** — Supervising the appointment schedule is one way to assure smooth patient flow. When you first begin the process, you may need to enlist the help of the clinical assistant or receptionist to understand each patient's need. Evaluate each appointment, approximately how long each appointment should take, and plan for contingencies that may arise. But remember that you cannot fully control this process.

Example: Two patients who each have complicated diagnoses are scheduled back-to-back; thus, there is the probability of the physician falling behind. Whenever possible, schedule such patients at the end of each session, i.e., one at the end of the morning; one at the end of the day.

- **Physician delays** — Have a contingency plan prepared when the physician is unavoidably detained (e.g., hospital rounds, surgery, etc.) Notify the patients immediately; do not make them wait 30 to 40 minutes. A patient considers her time as valuable as the physician does. Inform the patient of the anticipated delay and give him/her the option to reschedule.

  Telephone patients that are scheduled for the remainder of the morning or afternoon and let them know they may be delayed. The patient may choose to delay his/her arrival time or reschedule the appointment to another day.

- **Planning for the next day** — At the end of each day, the clinical assistant should review the charts of all the patients scheduled the next day. If laboratory tests, radiology exams or other procedures were ordered on the previous visit, the assistant should make sure that the test results are in the chart. If the physician has indicated that a procedure will be performed in the office on the scheduled visit, the assistant should make certain all necessary instruments are sterilized and readily available.

  The end of day chart review helps prevent delays by preplanning — anticipating procedure schedules and preparing the procedure room in advance with necessary instruments, sterilized and readily available.

  Generally, a physician spends a good part of the patient encounter searching the patient's chart for a lab test or X-ray report. For maximum efficiency, all records should be organized and compiled in a consistent format. A multi-division chart with metal fasteners, where all the patient's medical information is chronologically filed, makes information easier to find. Charts with metal fasteners increase security by eliminating misplaced or lost documents. A suggested organization plan is:

  - File progress notes in the *first section*.

  - File X-ray and lab reports in the *second section*.

  - File hospital notes in a *third section*.

  Studies show that compartmentalized charts save the physician at least five minutes during every encounter. Fasteners enable you to organize and keep the contents of your patient folder in a standardized sequence for the fastest finding and updating. Structure and documentation of medical records are discussed at length in Chapter 7.

- **Summary Report** — Provide the physician with a one-page summary report of the practice's vital statistics at the end of each month.   A monthly summary gives the physician concise data about the practice activity, and it can be reviewed in ten minutes or less. File the reports in a three-ring binder so that they may be reviewed and compared easily.

  Monthly Statistics Report form is shown as Exhibit 1.

- **Monthly Update** — Recording a monthly update on a cassette tape is another way to provide the physician with the month-end statistics. The physician can use commuting time to catch up on office news and practice data.

- **Patient Information Brochures** — Patient information brochures are another time saver. The practice needs an attractive, informative brochure that is given to each new patient and made available in the reception area. Patient information brochures can cut down on patient phone calls by 25 percent.

  In summary, regardless of what time management techniques you use, nothing takes the place of good, old-fashioned planning.

CHAPTER 2

Employee Relations

Statutes Overview

The administrator should have a working knowledge and a broad reference of all aspects of employment relations and the statutes that form the basis of all employment decisions. Following is a brief overview of laws governing the medical practice. Expanded information is provided on selected statutes thought to be of extreme risk and not easily understood.

Fair Labor Standards Act of 1938 (FLSA)

- Establishes minimum wage.

- Regulates child labor.

- Establishes overtime pay.

TIP: *Employees are entitled to overtime if they work more than 40 hours in a week. This includes working through their lunch — even if it is not a job requirement. Therefore, all overtime should be pre-approved.*

The FLSA requires employers to keep records on wages and hours worked. It is essential that you know and can prove the number of hours an employee works each week. Employee compensation should be on record, supported by time cards. The maintenance of this type of documentation facilitates accurate payment for overtime services and adheres to wage and hour laws.

The Department of Labor does not require a special format for wage records as long as they are easily ascertainable. Wage records should include:

- The employee's full name as used in Social Security records.

- The employee's Social Security Number, employee number or symbol, as used in payroll records.

- The employee's home address, including ZIP code.

- The employee's date of birth, if the employee is under the age of 19.

- The employee's sex.

- The employee's position.

- The time of the day and the day of the week when the employee's work begins.

- The regular hourly rate of pay.

- The amount and type of pay for any pay that is not included in the "regular rate."

- The hours worked by the employee on each work day, and the total hours for the week.

- The employee's total daily or weekly earnings (not including any premiums paid for overtime).

- The employee's total payment of overtime for the work week.

- Total wages for the employee for each pay period.

- The date of each payment made to the employee and the pay period covered by the payment.

- The total amount of additions to or deductions from wages for each pay period.

- For each deduction, the employer must show the following:
  - date
  - amount
  - nature of the deduction

Regardless of whether you use time clocks or time sheets, the important point is to maintain records of employees' work hours for a minimum of three years.

A work week is defined as 168 hours during seven consecutive 24-hour periods. It may begin on any day of the week. Each work week stands alone. There can be no averaging of two or more work weeks.

Employees must be paid for all hours worked in a work week. In general, "hours worked" includes all time an employee must be on duty, or on the employer's premises or in any other prescribed place of work. Also included is any additional time the employee is required or permitted to work. Overtime pay must be paid at a rate of at least one and one half times the regular rate of pay.

TIP: *"Overtime pay" is not paid for extra hours worked during a week when the employee is out for sick leave or vacation time since the employee was not physically on the job. Overtime is paid for the hours that exceed 40 hours.*

When violations are found or reported, the enforcement division of the FLSA is required to carry out an investigation and gather data on wages, hours, and other employment conditions or practices.

Willful violation can carry a fine up to $10,000. The Secretary of Labor may bring suit against the employer on behalf of the employee or the employee may bring a private suit. The employee is entitled to all back pay due as well as an additional amount equal to the back wages for "liquidated damages."

A two-year statute of limitations applies to recovery of back pay.

Equal Pay Act of 1963

- Amendment to Fair Labor Standards Act of 1938.

- Prohibits wage differential for men and women for jobs that require equal skills, effort, and responsibility when performed under similar working conditions.

The Civil Rights Act of 1964, Title VII

- Prohibits employment discrimination because of race, color, religion, sex, or national origin.

- Created the Equal Employment Opportunity Commission (EEOC) to enforce the act.

  (Expanded discussion follows in this chapter.)

Age Discrimination in Employment Act of 1967 (ADEA)

- Prohibits discrimination against persons aged 40 and older.

- Abolishes mandatory retirement at age 65.

  (Expanded discussion follows in this chapter.)

Equal Employment Opportunity Act of 1972

- Gives the EEOC the authority to institute legal action involving employment discrimination.

Pregnancy Discrimination Act of 1978

- States that discrimination on the basis of pregnancy, childbirth, or related medical condition constitutes unlawful sex discrimination.

TIP: *An applicant who is pregnant must be given the same consideration as other applicants.*

Consolidated Omnibus Budget Reconciliation Act of 1985 (COBRA)

- This federal law requires employers of 20 or more employees to offer employees and their dependents certain health insurance continuation rights if the employee is terminated, laid off, or has his hours reduced so that he no longer meets the eligibility requirements for health insurance coverage. (Expanded discussion follows in this chapter.)

Americans with Disabilities Act of 1990 (ADA)

- The employment provision of the ADA became effective July 26, 1992. On that date, employers with 25 or more employees were affected by the ADA. On July 26, 1994, the threshold level for coverage dropped to 15 or more employees.

- The ADA protects disabled persons from discrimination in employment, public services, public accommodations, and telecommunications.

  (Expanded discussion follows in this chapter.)

Family Medical Leave Act of 1993

- Affects employers with 50 or more employees within a 75-mile radius.

- Allows for 12 weeks of unpaid leave for qualified employees with no loss of benefit for the following reasons:
    - The birth, adoption, or foster care placement of a child.
    - To care for a child, spouse, or parent who has a serious health condition requiring personal care.
    - A serious health condition that causes the employee to be unable to perform the essential functions of the job.

Occupational Laws

Workers' Compensation Law

Workers' Compensation is governed almost entirely by state rather than federal law. The purpose of the Workers' Compensation system is to provide a uniform method of compensating employees for on-the-job injuries at a cost that is evenly distributed through insurance or other assessments against employers. Points to remember are:

- Request all information provided by your state's Workers' Compensation Board.

- Post the required information as directed.

- Update and keep records of claims.

TIP: *The required information must be posted in a place that is accessible and in full view of all employees. The break room is an excellent location. Include a checklist for handling an accident.*

Workers' Compensation Law is often ignored or forgotten by management once the required information has been posted. However, workplace injuries are increasing, and it is important that supervisors know the steps to follow if an employee is injured on the job.

Most states require employers to comply with the Workers' Compensation Law in one of two ways:

- Purchasing Workers' Compensation Insurance through a qualified carrier or a state insurance fund.

- Becoming self-insured by a process prescribed under state law.

Employers that fail to purchase insurance or obtain self-insurance approval lose the immunity normally afforded employers under the Workers' Compensation Law. Answering the following questions will provide a guide for steps to be taken in the event of an injury.

- Have you established a safety policy? A written policy develops employee awareness and expresses to all employees the intent to provide a safe workplace. Establishing a safe working environment can include posted signs, written rules, standard job procedures, personal protective equipment requirements, compliance with equipment codes, and rules for disposal of hazardous waste. Common steps in a safety program include:

- Remove the hazard, if possible.

- If the hazard cannot be removed, guard against it.

- If it cannot be effectively guarded, use personal protective equipment to protect employees from the hazard.

- Supervise and train employees to work safely and to be aware of the risks.

- Complete the *Employee Safety Orientation Checklist/Injury and Illness Prevention* for each employee. (See Exhibit 2-1.)

- Do you know the name of your Workers' Compensation Insurance carrier, the claims process, and the benefits involved?

- Do you have First Report of Injury forms or do you know your carrier's procedures (i.e., telephone reporting procedures)?

TIP: *Know your carrier's procedures for reporting claims.*

- Does every manager and supervisor in your practice know how to administer first aid?

- Do all employees know where to report injuries?

- Is every accident and injury investigated?

- Do all employees know who the practice's medical provider is?
(See *Dual Capacity Doctrine* below.)

- If your state permits you to direct an injured employee to a selected provider, do the employees know which providers you prefer? Our medical provider panel is:

____

____

____

____

____

____

TIP: *Know your state's requirements for choosing a panel of medical providers.*

- Is your Workers' Compensation policy aimed at getting the employee back to work?

- Are return-to-work goals stated on every claim you file?

- Are injured employees kept working on the job site whenever possible, even if in a lesser capacity or role?

- Do you visit the injured person on a regular basis to provide support and offer assistance?

- Do you know what to say and do when you visit an injured employee?

Dual Capacity Doctrine

This doctrine is sometimes used against medical employers that treat their own employees. If an employee is injured by an employer acting in the role of a third-party provider of medical services, the provider may be liable for injuries that result from the medical treatment. Although an accident may occur on the premises of a qualified medical provider, because of exposure to liability risks under the dual capacity doctrine, another provider should render medical care for an on-the-job injury. Therefore, after the injured employee receives first aid, the employee should receive medical attention from a prearranged provider. A physician should not enter into the dual role of employer and physician to the employee. The practice administrator or the physician should choose a medical provider that he would personally consult.

Use these steps to develop a plan for responding to a Workers' Compensation injury in your practice.

Immediately Follow the Steps Listed under Handling an Accident.

- **Handling an Accident**
  - Respond quickly and administer first aid.
  - Determine if the injury is covered by Workers' Compensation.
  - Accompany the injured worker to a selected medical provider.
  - Report the accident within the practice (to physician or practice administrator).
  - File an accident report. Report the injury to the Workers' Compensation Insurance carrier using the First Report of Injury forms. This is required by law.
  - Notify the family.

- **First Day**
  - Follow up with the employee.
  - Conduct an accident investigation. Consider every injury legitimate. (See *Accident/Injury Report* – Exhibit 2-2, 2-3 & 2-4.)
  - Counsel the employee and/or family on claims procedures, available benefits and the practice's continuing interest in the employee's welfare. (It is important for the administrator to have a working knowledge of Workers' Compensation procedures and benefits.)

- **Continuing involvement is the key to controlling claims**
  - Typically, it is the employee who is ignored by the employer who seeks an attorney to help get the benefits to which he or she is entitled.
  - Communicate continued concern for the employee's well being.

TIP: Keep the employee informed about his/her rights under Workers' Compensation.

- **First Week**
  - Make sure the insurer has contacted the employee about benefits and payment.
  - Talk to the treating physician to learn the diagnosis and treatment plan.

  – Develop a return-to-work plan. Can the employee accept a light duty assignment?

  – Stay in touch with the injured employee.

■ **First Month**

  – Calls, letters, and visits reinforce concern.

  – Stay in touch with the treating physician for updates on the employee's condition and any changes in treatment or diagnosis.

OSHA Work Place Requirements

The Occupational Safety & Health Administration (OSHA) was enacted in 1970 to ensure "safe and healthful working conditions" for employees. OSHA requirements imposed on employers are found in regulations and safety standards issued through the Secretary of Labor.

Medical employers have unique concerns for employee health and safety. The practice administrator has specific responsibility if an employee is exposed to a bloodborne pathogen or other potentially hazardous material. Train employees to follow the *Exposure Incident Protocol* (Exhibit 2-5). Complete an *Employee Safety Orientation Checklist/Injury and Illness Prevention* on each employee. This form should be a part of the office's procedure manual. The administrator should personally complete, or supervise the completion of the *Exposure Incident Form* (Exhibit 2-6) if an incident occurs. In addition to the incident report, the administrator should also complete or supervise the completion of a *Post-Exposure Incident Form.*
(See Exhibit 2-7.)

See forms provided in Exhibits section.

Labor Laws

Consolidated Omnibus Budget Reconciliation Act of 1985 (COBRA)

This federal law requires employers of 20 or more employees to offer employees and their dependents certain health insurance continuation rights if the employee is terminated, laid off, or has his or her hours reduced so that he or she no longer meets the eligibility requirements for health insurance coverage. If any of those events occur, the employee or dependents can choose to continue health care coverage for 18 months at the employer's group premium rate (plus two percent for administrative costs). Only employees who are terminated due to gross misconduct (behavior that amounts to a crime) can be denied these health insurance continuation rights.

Certain other events, such as an employee's death, divorce or legal separation, trigger health insurance continuation rights on the part of the employee's dependents for up to 36 months.

If an employer fails to comply with COBRA requirements, the employer, among other sanctions, may lose its income tax deduction for the expenses for its group health plan.

TIP: The practice administrator's responsibility is to send any eligible, terminated employee a letter notifying him of his COBRA benefits.

Sexual Harassment

Sexual harassment includes unwelcome sexual advances, requests for sexual favors, and other verbal or physical conduct of a sexual nature. The guidelines state that such conduct violates Title VII of the Civil Rights Act of 1964 when:

- Submission to such conduct is made a term or condition of an individual's employment.

- Submission to or rejection of such conduct is used as the basis for employment decisions affecting an individual (e.g., denial of a pay increase, promotion, transfer, leave of absence, imposing disciplinary action, promising to withhold disciplinary action, etc.).

- Such conduct interferes with performance or creates an offensive environment.

Title VII places responsibility of the employer for the conduct of others:

- **Supervisors.** The employer is liable for the acts of its officers, agents and supervisors with respect to sexual harassment regardless of whether the employer knew or should have known about the unlawful conduct.

- **Actions of Non-Supervisory Employees.** The employer is responsible for the acts of sexual harassment occurring between fellow employees where the employer, its agent or supervisors knew or should have known about the unlawful conduct, unless the employer can show that it took "immediate and appropriate corrective action." The guidelines do not define what is meant by "immediate and appropriate corrective action."

- **Actions of Non-Employees.** The employer is also liable for the actions of non-employees (e.g., patients, outside sales representatives, contractors, delivery personnel, etc.) with respect to sexual harassment in the work place where the employer knew or should have known of the conduct and failed to take immediate and appropriate corrective action.

The employer is responsible for taking *preventative actions* to avoid sexual harassment. Suggested actions are:

- Raising the subject of sexual harassment with the work force and expressing strong disapproval.

- Developing appropriate sanctions and penalties when unlawful conduct is committed.

- Advising employees of their right to raise and how to raise sexual harassment claims under Title VII.

- Developing methods to sensitize all concerned.

Sexual Harassment is defined broadly by Title VII guidelines. The range of conduct that may be viewed as unlawful may vary widely with the sensitivity of the individual.

Responsive Actions of Employers are:

- Adopt and publicize to all employees a written policy statement that prohibits sexual harassment in the work place.

- Adopt an in-house complaint resolution procedure.

- Fully and promptly investigate sexual harassment complaints.

- Explain the policies to staff members.

The liability imposed upon employers for sexual harassment suggests that special efforts must be exerted to minimize the legal risk. Title VII prohibits employers from retaliating against an employee for the employee's opposition to an unlawful employment practice or for asserting any rights granted under the Civil Rights Act.

TIP: Generally, employees do not fully understand the far-reaching ramifications of sexual harassment. Conduct an in-service training session for all employees to explain your in-house complaint and resolution procedures. Answer any concerns employees may have.

Americans With Disabilities Act (ADA)

The Americans with Disabilities Act protects disabled persons from discrimination in employment, public services, public accommodations, and telecommunications. The employment provisions of the ADA became effective July 26, 1992. Employers with 15 or more employees are affected by this Act as of July 26, 1994.

- **Anti-Discrimination Provisions.** The law prohibits covered employers from discriminating against a "qualified individual with a disability." With respect to an individual, a "disability" means:

  > "A physical or mental impairment that substantially limits one
  > or more of the major life activities of such individual..."

  A physical or mental impairment means any physiological disorder or condition, cosmetic disfigurement, or anatomical loss affecting most body systems, and mental or psychological disorders such as mental illness, learning disabilities, mental retardation, etc. It includes HIV infection and AIDS.

  A person who has been successfully rehabilitated and who no longer uses illegal drugs or abuses alcohol is considered a person with a disability and thus is protected by the ADA. (Current use of alcohol that prevents an individual from performing his/her duties is not protected.)

A "qualified individual with a disability" is defined as "an individual with a disability who, with or without reasonable accommodation, can perform the essential functions of the employment position that such individual holds or desires." If an employer has prepared a written job description before advertising or interviewing applicants for the job, this job description will be considered evidence of the essential functions of the job. If, for example, a person in a wheelchair applies for a switchboard operator position, the essential function being to answer the telephone, his or her disability has no relevance in assessing the individual's qualifications for that job. The same is not true if the person is deaf and applies for that position.

- **Reasonable Accommodation.** The ADA requires an employer to make "reasonable accommodation" for an individual's disability. The employer need not incur "undue hardship," however. Reasonable accommodation may include:

  - Making existing facilities readily accessible to and usable by the disabled.

  - Job restructuring.

  - Part-time or modified work schedules.

  - Reassignment to a vacant position.

- Acquisition or modification of equipment or devices.

- Appropriate adjustment or modifications of examinations, training materials, or policies.

- The provision of qualified readers or interpreters.

- Other similar accommodations.

TIP: *In a leased space, both the lessee and lessor are responsible for making the premises accessible to the disabled.*

Whether an action is a "reasonable accommodation" or an "undue hardship" will depend upon the particular circumstances. Factors that will be considered are:

- The overall financial resources of the employer.

- The overall size of the business with respect to the number of employees and the number, type, and location of its facilities.

- The type of operation maintained, including the composition, structure, and functions of the entire work force.

- The nature and cost of the accommodations needed.

TIP: *An example of "reasonable accommodation" is the installation a bell or buzzer at the door of the building to alert someone that a disabled person needs help. An "undue hardship" is installing an elevator in a two-story building where only stairs exist.*

While it is clear that more is required than a minimal effort or expenditure, the type of effort or expenditure will vary from case to case.

The ADA provides that an employer may not conduct medical examinations or make medical inquiries of a job applicant or employee about whether such applicant or employee is an individual with a disability or about the nature or severity of the disability unless the examination or inquiry is job-related and justified by business necessity.

- **Enforcement.** The ADA is enforced by the Equal Employment Opportunity Commission (EEOC) in the same manner as it enforces Title VII of the Civil Rights Act of 1964. The same remedies that apply to Title VII apply to the ADA. Currently those remedies include reinstatement, back pay, compensatory and punitive damages.

Age Discrimination in Employment Act (ADEA)

It is unlawful for an employer to discipline or discharge an employee who is over 40 because of the employee's age. The ADEA does not regulate job-related discipline. The purpose of the law is to eliminate discrimination in employment based simply on the fact that an employee (age 40 and over) is getting older. If an employee is no longer able to meet uniformly applied production standards, discipline or discharge is not unlawful.

- **Enforcement.** Enforcement of the Age Discrimination in Employment Act is the responsibility of the EEOC. Suits to enforce the law may be brought either by the individual employee or by the government and may result in back pay and reinstatement. An employer's willful violation of the Act could result in additional damages in an amount equal to the back pay, a fine of not more than $10,000, and imprisonment for up to six months.

Federal Record Keeping Requirements

The following is a list of the types and retention periods of records various federal laws require employers to keep.

Applications for Employment

- Required by Age Discrimination in Employment Act and Title VII, 1964 Civil Rights Act.
- One year.

Advertisements to Hire Employees

- Required by Age Discrimination in Employment Act.
- One year.

Certificates of Age

- Required by Fair Labor Standards Act.
- Duration of employment of individuals under the age of 18.

Discrimination Complaint Records and Actions

- Required by Title VII, the Age Discrimination in Employment Act of 1967, Rehabilitation Act, and Vietnam Era Veterans' Readjustment Assistance Act.
- Until final disposition.

ERISA Plan Disclosures; Annual Summaries and Annual Reports

- Required by ERISA.
- Six years after filing date.

Employment Contracts

- Required by Fair Labor Standards Act.
- Three years.

Employment History: Promotions, Demotions, Transfers, Layoffs, Terminations, Pay Rate, Training

- Required by the Title VII, Civil Rights Act of 1964, and the Age Discrimination in Employment Act.
- One year.

Hiring Requests to Employment Agencies

- Required by Title VII, Civil Rights Act of 1964, and the Age Discrimination in Employment Act.
- One year.

Immigration Documentation

- Required by Immigration Reform and Control Act (Form I-9).
- Three years from date of hire or one year from date of termination, whichever is later.

Injury Summary

- Required by Occupational Safety and Health Administration (OSHA Form 101).
- Three years.
- First aid records for injuries covering lost work time required for five years.

Medical Records

- Required by the Occupational Safety and Health Administration for employees with certain occupational exposures (including exposure to bloodborne pathogens).
- Duration of employment plus 30 years.

Order, Shipping, Billing, and Payment Records

- Required by the Fair Labor Standards Act.
- Three years.

Payroll Records

- Required by Fair Labor Standards Act, Child Labor Law, Equal Pay Act, Title VII, and Age Discrimination in Employment Act.
- Three years.

Physical Examination Results

- Required by Title VII and the Age Discrimination in Employment Act of 1967.
- One year.

Sale and Purchase Agreements

- Required by Fair Labor Standards Act.
- Three years.

Tests: Employer-Administered Aptitude or Other Employment Tests

- Required by Title VII and the Age Discrimination in Employment Act.
- One year.

Training Records

- Required by OSHA's Bloodborne Pathogens Standard.
- Three years.

Wage Records: Time Cards, Rate Tables, Work Schedules, Etc.

- Required by Fair Labor Standards Act and Equal Pay Act.
- Two years.

Wages Paid, Including Additions to or Deductions From Wages Paid

- Required by Fair Labor Standards Act.
- Three years.

Posting Requirements

Federal and state laws often require employers to post a notice about a particular law. These notices are usually provided in the form of posters or permits and should be posted in a conspicuous place easily accessible to all employees (i.e., the break room).

Listed below are the posters that employers are required to display under federal law. Not all are required of every employer. Refer to the specifications listed previously in this chapter to see if your practice qualifies.

- **Age Discrimination, Disability Discrimination, Equal Employment**
  - Poster titled "Equal Employment Opportunity is the Law."
  - Available from EEOC offices.

- **Child Labor, Minimum Wage and Overtime**
  - Wage-hour poster 1088 (Federal Minimum Wage).
  - Available from the U.S. Department of Labor.

- **Family and Medical Leave**
  - Poster required by Family and Medical Leave Act of 1993.
  - Available from the U.S. Department of Labor.

- **Polygraph Testing**
  - Wage-hour poster 1462 (Employee Polygraph Protection Act) required.
  - Available from the U.S. Department of Labor.

- **Safety**
  - OSHA poster 2203 (Job Safety & Health Protection) required.
  - Available from the U.S. Department of Labor.
  - OSHA also requires posting an annual summary of job injuries (OSHA Form 200).

The posters may be obtained from the government agency charged with enforcing a particular law. Most agencies have developed a single poster that satisfies the requirements of several different laws administered by that agency. There are also private companies that publish posters that employers are required to have.

Contact the following agencies to obtain these posters:

> Equal Employment Opportunity Poster Office
> 2401 E. Street N.W.
> Washington, D.C. 20507

> U. S. Department of Labor Posters
> 200 Constitution Ave. N.W., Room S-3502
> Washington, D.C. 20210

Employment Categories

The administrator should become familiar with the laws governing work hours and wage payments, including minimum wages, overtime, deductions from wage, and child labor. Refer to the Fair Labor Standards Act (FLSA) to obtain a working knowledge of this national policy on minimum wages and overtime payments. (See Chapter 2, Page 21.) This complex law determines whether an employer is subject to federal minimum wage and overtime requirements. Most medical employees are covered. First, ascertain the status of your practice. Then, conclude the exempt or nonexempt status of each employee.

- **■ *Exempt.*** The following employment categories have been adapted for application to the medical practice for defining employees who are ***exempt*** from overtime pay requirements.

  An ***Executive Employee*** must meet all of the following definitions to be exempt: (Practice Administrators are typically considered exempt.)

  - Primary duty consists of the management of the practice or a customarily recognized department.

  - Must supervise at least two full-time employees.

  - Must have authority to hire and fire or to recommend those actions.

  - Must regularly exercise discretionary powers.

  - Must spend no more than 20 percent of working hours on non-managerial duties.

  An ***Administrative Employee*** must meet the following definitions to be exempt: (Administrative assistants, personnel directors, office managers, and laboratory supervisors are typically considered exempt.)

  - Primary duty must be responsible office or non-manual work directly related to management policy or general business operations.

  - Must regularly exercise discretion and independent judgment. Must have authority to make important decisions.

  - Must assist the executive.

  - Must not spend more than 20 percent of work week in non-administrative duties.

  A ***Professional Employee*** must meet all the following requirements to be exempt: (Physicians, registered nurses, registered or certified medical technologists, physician assistants, speech pathologists, and physical therapists are typically considered exempt.)

  - Primary duty must be work requiring knowledge of an advanced type in a field of science, usually obtained by a prolonged course of specialized instruction and study.

  - Must consistently exercise discretion and judgment.

  - Must do work that is mainly intellectual and varied.

  - Must not spend more than 20 percent of work week on activities not a part of or incident to professional duties.

  Nonexempt. Among common positions that typically are considered ***nonexempt*** are the following:

  - Licensed practical nurses.

  - Nurse's aides.

    – Laboratory technicians or assistants.

    – Clerical workers.

    – Orderlies.

    – Food service employees.

    – Janitorial employees.

At-Will Contracts

The most common type of employment agreement in the health care industry is an oral, "at-will" agreement. This establishes a relationship in which the employer and employee work at the will of the other. The practice administrator must understand this relationship.

- **Concept.** Just as an employee can resign at any time, so can the employer terminate the employee at any time for any reason.

- **Exceptions.** "At-will" does not apply to a job in which a contract is in effect stating a specific period of employment. The right of the employer to apply the "at-will" doctrine does not override the restrictions placed on the employer such as the discriminations defined in Title VII of the 1964 Civil Rights Act.

By using the term "at-will" versus "just cause," an employee serves at the discretion of the medical practice and therefore may be dismissed with or without cause. Utilization of the term "just cause" sets a prerequisite that justifiable cause must be shown in order to discharge an employee.

TIP: *Use specific language in your employee handbook to indicate that employees of your practice are employees "at-will."*

CHAPTER 3

Personnel Management

Hiring Only the Best

The hiring of dedicated, efficient employees should begin before the actual need to recruit arises. Assess your practice's long- and short-term needs. Do not wait until a position is open before you develop the job description or candidate profile. Anticipate future needs and have a network of contacts to call upon when a position must be filled.

Develop a recruitment process.

Here are some tips:

- Develop a network with other practice administrators. Join professional societies and the Chamber of Commerce and attend the meetings and networking luncheons. These activities will furnish you with contacts that can help you locate potential employees when the need arises.

- Talk to supply vendors and pharmaceutical representatives who are in physician's offices every day. Ask if they have heard of offices that are down-sizing or if they know of employees looking for other opportunities.

- Offer a recruitment bonus of $100 to any employee who identifies a qualified candidate that you hire and who remains with the practice for six months or longer. A member of your staff is apt to recognize a candidate who fits in with your practice.

- To gain valuable insight into hiring a new employee, conduct an exit interview with the departing employee.

- Follow a timetable for recruiting a new employee. *Do without until you find the right candidate!*

Preparing the Job Description

Job descriptions can be prepared in a variety of formats, but typically include the following elements:

- *Job Title.* The name of the job.

- *Job Summary.* A one, or two sentence summary that defines the overall function of the job.

- *Job Qualification.* A brief listing of educational and experience qualifications needed to perform the job.

- *Duties and Responsibilities.* A list of major job tasks listing what is to be accomplished by the employee.

(See *Sample Job Descriptions* — Exhibits 3-1, 3-2, 3-3.)

Using Job Descriptions

The job description is a useful management tool that helps promote good employee relations and makes the administrator's job much easier. When jobs are defined, the administrator has a handy reference for dealing with many personnel management tasks that arise.

- **Defining Job Relationships.** Job descriptions help clarify how each job interacts with other jobs by defining nature of contacts, authority, and supervision given or received.

- **Training and Orientation of New Workers.** The job description provides a ready-made outline to orient the new employee to job responsibilities. Training for employees on work procedures or job skills can also be developed based upon the job description.

- **Communication of Job Responsibilities.** Throughout the employment relationship, a job description serves as the standard of reference for defining the employee's job responsibilities. A properly prepared job description is the supervisor's best defense against the employee who tries to shirk an assignment by saying, "That's not my job."

- **Recruiting and Selecting.** The job description can be an invaluable aid in recruiting and selecting new employees. Job description details are useful in specifying work qualifications, in evaluating resumés or applications, and in determining interview questions. According to the Americans with Disabilities Act of 1990, an employee's written job description, prepared before advertising or interviewing for the job, is considered evidence of the essential functions of the job. They may be used for determining reasonable accommodation under the ADA.

- **Appraising Performance.** The job description provides a ready list of what tasks the employee should be performing. Referring to the job description, the supervisor can then rate how well the employee performs assigned tasks.

- **Wage-Hour Law Compliance.** The job description is an important basis for documenting job responsibilities to classify jobs as exempt from federal and state wage-hour laws. The Fair Labor Standards Act, for example, exempts executive, professional, administrative, and outside sales positions from minimum wage, overtime pay, and time keeping requirements. Nonexempt employees, such as licensed practical nurses, nurse's aides, laboratory technicians or assistants, clerical workers, etc., are covered by the FLSA.

- **Pay Determination.** Human resources and compensation specialists use job descriptions to determine pay structures and pay ranges for jobs. Job descriptions are an important basis for comparing practice pay rates to area salary surveys to assure that pay levels are competitive.

Create a Candidate Profile

To create a candidate profile, you may want to begin with these considerations.

- **Education.** What level of education will the candidate need to successfully handle the job? Will a high school diploma suffice, or will the candidate need an accounting background?

- **Skills.** What type of office machines should the candidate be familiar with? Will computer word processing or spreadsheet experience be required? The training process is reduced if the candidate is familiar with the software programs you use.

- **Experience.** What experience is required for the position being filled? Experience with coding, medical terminology and claims filing are necessary to the insurance billing position, but medical office experience may not be required for a file clerk.

- **Licensing.** Does the physician prefer an LPN or RN? Will procedures be performed that require some level of licensure, i.e., chemotherapy?

- **Specialized Training.** An employee hired to perform simple lab tests or X-rays may not require a license, but the proper candidate will need some sort of special training.

Place the Advertisement

Advertisements for any position must be carefully written to avoid any appearance of discrimination against either gender, age, race, religion, national origin or disability. The ad should tell enough about the job to interest prospective applicants. List the minimal educational requirements, work experience and skill levels that are acceptable. Focus on what the job requires rather than the type of person you prefer. However, before you go to the expense of placing a newspaper or journal advertisement, consult with professional associates for names of potential applicants. Ask other practice administrators for resumés they have on file. Ask them to send you resumés of applicants they interviewed but elected not to hire. Always ask why they did not select a particular candidate. A highly qualified candidate may not have suited their needs but may be a perfect fit for a position in your office.

When advertising, have candidates send their written or typed resumés to a box number instead of listing the practice's telephone number and office address. This will allow you to select the most qualified applicants without speaking to all those who answer the ad.

Review the Resumés

Remember that resumés are simply a synopsis of what the applicant wants you to know about them. Taken at face value, resumés can be misleading. Develop the ability to read between the lines.

- **Experience** is a plus in most any position; however, frequent job changes may indicate problems. Job changing is a positive indication if:

  - Each new position had increasing responsibility and reimbursement.

  - New skills were added within the candidate's field.

  - The candidate has an insatiable desire to learn.

  On the other hand, job changing is a negative indication if:

  - It reveals a lack of dedication and commitment.

  - Each new position has been a repeat of the old, in several different offices, at the same or slightly more pay.

  - If the applicant only changes jobs for more money.

- **Education.** How important is education? An extensive educational background often tells how much a candidate is willing to invest in his or her future.

  - How has the applicant's education translated into experience and career choices?

  - Has the candidate continued to learn through continuing education courses?

  - Is the candidate's education relevant to the industry today?

- ***Personal Interests.*** What do personal interests tell you?

  - Varsity letters may indicate that the applicant is a high energy person who is also competitive and aggressive. This may not be what you need for a receptionist or an accounts coordinator, but may be an ideal characteristics for a leadership role.

  - Are sports interests for individual sports or team sports? These give clues about teamwork abilities versus solo assignments.

  - Has the applicant been a team captain or team leader? These roles prepare individuals for supervisory positions.

All resumés should be retained for at least a year. Avoid making notes of any kind on the resumé or on the application form. If you are sending the resumé to be reviewed by the physician or another person in the office, write your comments on a separate piece of paper and route with the resumé.

Telephone Screening of Candidates

After you have reviewed the resumés, select three to five applicants to interview by phone. The objective of the telephone interview is to learn about the applicant's current status and timetable, to ascertain their reason for leaving current or previous position, and to discover their objectives in seeking employment in your office.

Prepare a list of questions to ask every candidate you screen. Asking the same questions allows you to compare "apples to apples." Be prepared to ask other questions in response to the candidates' answers.

Ask open-ended but explicit questions, such as, "What do you want in a job?" "What do you need in a job?" "Why are you leaving your present position?" "What particular skills or experience do you have that make you the best candidate for this position?"

Ask questions that will allow you to eliminate a candidate immediately. For example, ask the range of pay they need or expect. You may find they are priced out of your range. Remember, however, that does not mean they will not accept the position, if offered. They may be looking for a career change or location that is closer to their home.

Define the candidate's time frame for availability. Are they be able to begin work in two weeks, or is a thirty-day notice required?

Setting Appointments for Interviews

Once the telephone screening process is complete, there should be at least two or three candidates you wish to interview face to face. There are four objectives in conducting an interview. Advance preparation will enable you to accomplish these objectives.

- Gain a better understanding of the candidate.

- Tell the candidate about your practice and its goals.

- Determine if the candidate fits your needs.

- Determine if the practice fits the candidate's needs.

If you plan to have other employees involved in the interview process, it is best to have each one concentrate on a specific area. For example, if you are hiring an additional billing or insurance clerk, the incumbent employees should ask questions about coding and billing procedure to determine the candidate's knowledge and skill level.

Interviewing

Active listening is a critical factor in the interviewing process. It is a good rule of thumb to allot at least two-thirds of the interview time to listening. Once you have listened to the candidate describe his talents and accomplishments, ask some open-ended questions that relate specifically to the position to be filled.

Here are some examples of questions to ask candidates for a receptionist position.

- How do you answer the telephone in your current (most recent) job?

- How would you change this procedure?

- How many incoming lines did you answer?

- Did the practice have written protocol for answering the telephone?

- What was your procedure when a patient presented at the reception window?

- Was there a glass window opening to the reception area? Was it kept open or closed? How do you feel about the window?

- When a patient presents at the desk after his visit, what procedure did you go through?

These questions give valuable insight into the candidate's "people skills." The ability to solicit payment for services is dependent on an individual's personality and ease of talking with patients.

Also ask a series of questions about the physician for whom the candidate previously worked.

- What medical school did the physician attend?

- Was the physician board certified?

- What services did the practice offer?

Answers to these questions tell you how much the candidate knew about the practice and the physicians she worked for. You will also hear how patients' questions about the practice were answered.

Use the candidate's personal interests to attain insight into personality and learning ability. As an interviewing exercise, provide at least three books with different topics, such as a professional self-help book, a romance novel, and a biography of a famous person and/or a historical novel. Ask the candidate to choose the book she would prefer to read. Ask why it was chosen. There are no wrong choices. Each choice indicates a personality "type." Personality types can be helpful for matching candidates to the position.

If experience and education are equal, a candidate who reads extensively is usually the preferred choice.

A candidate who is interested in nutrition and exercise can be a good fit for a physician's office. Such individuals usually understand the importance of good health and have a high level of energy.

For certain positions, giving a brief proficiency test is appropriate. An employer is allowed to set certain standards for employees to perform the *essential* functions of the job. For example, you may require a transcriptionist to type 70 words per minute. You do not have to justify the reason or explain why 65 wpm is not good enough. If the applicant cannot type 70 wpm, the evaluation ends there. To avoid discrimination, give the same test to every applicant for that position.

Requiring an applicant to complete a coding quiz or solve a coding problem is an excellent way to test the skills for an insurance biller.

When testing, be sure that accommodations are made for a disabled candidate that will allow him to compete equally with an applicant who is not disabled. For example, if you are testing the keyboarding skills of a candidate in a wheelchair, be sure that the wheelchair fits comfortably under the desk and that the candidate is not restricted in any way. You may need to move the computer to an area that will better accommodate the wheelchair.

Federal discrimination laws also apply to hiring. In seeking information from an applicant, ask yourself:

- Is this a question I would ask either a man or a woman?

- Is this question really needed to judge an applicant's competence or qualifications for the job?

Questions relating to the following should be avoided.

- Age or date of birth

- Sex or race

- Birthplace or national origin

- Religion

- Place of residence

- Arrest and conviction record

- Military service

- Health or disabilities

- Height or weight

- Child care arrangements

The candidate should make a good visual impression. Consider if this person will fit your medical family. How is she dressed for the interview? Clinical personnel, particularly if dressed in uniforms, should be neat and clean in appearance. Nails should be short, without bright polish. Uniforms should appear white and not discolored. Overall appearance such as hair and make-up should be appropriate for a clinical atmosphere.

Checking References

Before you make a final selection of a candidate for any position, take the time to check references. Letters of reference may provide valuable insight, but they do not take the place of a thorough telephone conference with a prior employer.

Many companies have established a policy of giving only basic information about a past employee. Dates of employment, rate of pay and the position the employee held is usually all the information you will receive. This is when your networking can benefit you. Do you know someone who has previously worked with your candidate who will give you an informed reference?

Let the applicant know if you have been unable to get satisfactory reference information. Ask them for the names of additional references. When checking references, look for the following information.

- References should be current. It is best to contact someone with whom the applicant has worked within the last twelve to eighteen months. Rather than calling a reference that employed or worked with an applicant five years ago, ask the applicant for more recent references.

- If the applicant does not give a recent employer as a reference, ask for an explanation.

- Friends and family are not considered objective sources.

- Call at least three references.

- Always ask if the employee is eligible for re-hire.

Making the Offer

You have now reached the final phase of the hiring process. The offer should be made in writing with a place for the new employee to sign, indicating acceptance.

- Include a job description. All job offer letters should contain the following statement: *This letter is an offer of employment only and does not constitute a contract of any kind.*

- The offer letter should include the start date, the rate of pay on an hourly, weekly, or monthly basis. **Do not state the pay on an annual basis.** To do so may be viewed as a yearly contract. Indicate the hours the employee is expected to work and include any benefits that will be provided. Inform the employee of any dress code in effect in your practice or if she is expected to wear a uniform.

- Do not make any employment promises during the interview or the job offer process. Avoid statements such as:

  - You will not be fired without just cause.

  - You will be with us as long as you do your job.

  - You will have job security here.

  - There are no layoffs in this practice.

  - You will become a **permanent** employee after the probation period.

Once the offer letter has been signed by the prospective employee, a copy should be put into the employee's personnel file. *A sample offer letter is shown on page 43.*

Setting Up The Personnel File

Every employee should have a personnel file, including the physicians. Each file should contain the following documents and be maintained appropriately.

- **Personnel File Contents.** The typical file should contain all government-mandated forms and employee benefit enrollment forms, as applicable:

    - Resumé
    - Employment Application
    - Reference Checklist
    - W-4 Form
    - State Income Tax Form, if applicable
    - I-9 Form
    - Payroll Set-Up Form
    - Health Insurance Enrollment Form
    - Long-Term Disability Enrollment Form
    - 401(k) Enrollment Form
    - Flex Benefits Form
    - Personnel Policies Acknowledgement Form (Disclaimer)
    - Attendance Records
    - Employment Letter
    - Salary Change Sheet
    - Performance Reviews
    - Warning or Disciplinary Letters
    - New Employee Checklist
    - Training Checklist

- **Employer Access and Retention.** Personnel files should be kept in a locked cabinet, accessed only by designated employee responsible for their maintenance.

- **Employee Access.** The employee has the right to access his file at any time, in the presence of a designated employee.

- **Retention.** The file should be retained for three years following termination.

- **Explanation of Benefits (EOBs)** from the health care plan are not filed in the personnel file. They are placed in a locked file and may only be accessed by the employee in the presence of a designated employee.

The Probationary Period

When hiring, notify the new employee that she will be working within a ninety-day probationary period. Use this time for orientation and training.   During this period, the administrator should monitor the employee's attitude, work habits and capabilities and assure that she is receiving the proper instructions.

The employee or the employer may end the employment relationship "at-will" at any time during this probationary period, with or without cause, and without advance notice.

Employees will assume "regular" status upon satisfactory completion of the probationary period.

On the first day, present the employee with a copy of the The Employee Handbook. Take time to explain the basic work rules and regulations including:

- Compensation and benefits

- Payroll deductions

- Vacation schedules and sick leave

- Safety and health

Help the employee have a global view of the practice and see how his/her job fits into the overall plan. This explanation will emphasize of the importance of the new employee's role and will encourage pride in the job and the practice.

Ask the employee to read The Employee Handbook. Offer to answer any questions about policy and procedures. Address any tentative issues such as dress codes, overtime, etc. After the Handbook has been reviewed, the employee should sign an acknowledgement form. Place a copy of the acknowledgement form in the personnel file.

Credentialing of Health Care Providers

All physicians must be credentialed annually to maintain hospital privileges. The practice administrator is generally called on to ensure that the necessary paperwork for credentialing or recredentialing is received by the hospital.

With the insurgence of mid-level providers in the medical practice such as physician's assistants and nurse practitioners, it is recommended that every practice have a process in place for screening future and current licensed employees — even if they have been subjected to hospital credentialing.

It is also wise to check the credentials of any independent contractor or locum tenens you may use in the practice. Use the following list to assure that you have done a thorough job of checking the credentials of any physician or licensed employee who works in the practice.

- Verify education and training.

- Keep a current copy of each employee/physician's professional license.

- Check employment history and obtain letters of reference.

- Check for license suspensions, revocations or application denials in current and prior resident states.

- Verify liability coverage and tail coverage.

- Assure that the employee's limits of liability insurance are adequate for:
  - Hospital coverage
  - State requirements
  - Practice requirements

Hiring Independent Contractors

Individuals hired as independent contractors (IC) are usually physician's assistants, nurse practitioners, or other professional licensed individuals.

Sometimes an independent contractor is hired for short-term projects or to cover vacation or sick leave for a regular employee. These short-term agreements usually do not present any legal or tax problems. However, if the IC will be working in the practice on a regular basis, make sure you are in compliance with the Internal Revenue Service. The following guidelines determine if someone is an employee or an independent contractor.

- A person is considered an employee if:
    - You control how she does the work.
    - You determine the work hours.
    - The IC is not available for work in other offices.
    - You supply all the equipment to do the job.
    - He could walk away, leaving you no recourse.
- There are four ways to prove a worker is truly independent.
    - If the IC bills you periodically on his own stationery.
    - If the bills are for varying amounts. A standard weekly or monthly fee may sound like a salary.
    - If some of his work is done on his own premises.
    - If the IC is incorporated. This alone may be enough to satisfy the IRS.

The IRS and many state agencies are quite aggressive in pursuing employees who try to avoid taxes by characterizing employees as independent contractors. Avoid liability by properly classifying your employees.

Outsourcing/Employee Leasing

Medical practices have been outsourcing functions such as billing and collections or medical transcription for a number of years. Employee leasing, however, is a relatively new idea. The outsourcing company employs the staff, contracts with the physician for the provision of the staff, pays the staff and provides benefits.

There are many advantages to employee leasing. Some physicians are more than happy to turn over the time-consuming, administrative hassles of interviewing and hiring new staff. Leasing also limits the dealing with difficult employees on issues such as vacation, sick leave, and promotions. Concerns about discrimination and personnel policies are also minimized.

It is important to remember, however, that the employees are not completely under the control of the practice. They may not be as friendly with the patients, or as cooperative with the physician. You will need to consider both the tangible and intangible benefits and disadvantages as part of your decision to outsource. Consider the cost of performing these functions in-house as opposed to outsourcing.

Sample Job Offer Letter

Dear ___________________,

Medical Practice Associates is pleased to offer you the position of Medical Assistant. If you
accept our employment offer, your effective date of employment will be ________________.
Your work hours will be from 8:00 a.m. to 5:00 p.m., Monday through Friday.

As we discussed, your rate of pay will be _______________ per hour. Our pay periods are on
the first and fifteenth of each month.

During your first day we will discuss health insurance and other practice benefits, fill out the
necessary tax forms, and review your job description.

This letter is an offer of employment only and does not constitute a contract of any kind. The
employee and employer agree that the employment is for an indefinite period of time and
employment may be terminated at any time and for any reason by either party.

We look forward to your acceptance and having you on our medical team!

Sincerely,

Shirley Bragg
Practice Administrator
Medical Practice Associates

Please indicate your response to this offer by signing and and returning this
letter by __________________.

____
Accepted   Date

Orientation and Training

Hiring and training new employees is one of the most expensive processes in a medical office. Your employees are your most valuable asset. It makes good sense to properly integrate them into the practice and give them the proper training.

The orientation process begins on the first day the employee begins work. Set the new employee's arrival time on their first day an hour or so after the office opens. This will allow you time to start your day and take care of any issues that are important before you sit down with the new person.

When the new employee arrives, set aside at least an hour of your time to meet with him. Allow a ten-minute break in the appointment schedule for the new employee to tour the office and meet each physician and employee.

It also works well if you cut off patient appointments at 3:30 or 4:00 p.m. on the day before the new-hire starts. Have him come in for an informal welcome reception. Serve light refreshments, such as cookies and coffee or soft drinks. This way you can make your introductions to physicians and staff at the end of the day when the schedule is finished and while there are no patients waiting. Present the new employee with a name badge to make them an "official" member of the team. This makes the new employee feel welcome and gives them a feeling of joining a team. You may also wish to begin orientation at this time. Since other employees will be going home, you will have no interruptions as you begin the orientation process.

Show the new employee his work station and provide a thorough overview of the following:

- The employer physician's philosophies of the medical practice and the history of the practice.

- Any future plans for the practice, such as bringing in new physicians or adding new services.

- A copy of the physician's Curriculum Vitae for familiarity with the physician's training and background.

- The services offered within the practice. What procedures the physician performs.

- All ancillary services that the practice provides.

- An employee roster that lists each employee's name and the position they hold.

- The probationary period and how it works. Explain that they will be receiving close supervision and help during this time.

Training for the New Position

Now that you have introduced the employee to the rest of the team, begin the training process. A few words of caution are in order here. Be careful not to overload the new employee with too much information at once. A ten-day training schedule is recommended, followed by ten days of observation.

- The first five days of the training period should consist mainly of observing the person who is currently doing the job. If the new employee is replacing an employee who has already left the practice, it will probably become the administrator's role to train the new person. If the training is delegated to another employee, the administrator must work closely with the trainer to assure that thorough training is provided.

- During the second week, or about the sixth day, the new employee should begin to perform the job functions while being observed by and receiving feedback from the trainer.

- On or about the seventh day, the trainer should allow the new employee to handle all the routine functions of the job. Remain close by to assist if a problem arises.

- If a good hiring decision has been made and the training has been properly conducted, the new employee should be working independently by the third week.

- During the remainder of the probationary period, continue to provide support to the new employee. Be lavish in your encouragement and quick to provide additional training, as appropriate.

- If it is clear that the employee is not going to work out, do not delay the inevitable. If you are convinced that adequate training has been provided, discharging the employee at this time is best for both parties.

Final Training Tips

- Hire the right person; initial selection is critical. Take the time to do a thorough job of recruiting and interviewing.

- Start the training early. If the new employee is a replacement, it is best to bring them aboard at least two weeks before the incumbent employee leaves.

- Provide regular instruction. Remember not to overload the employee with too much information at one time. Short training sessions are preferred to all-day marathons.

- Assure frequent communication. Set aside specific times during the day to check on or meet with the new recruit. He should not have to "run you down" to ask questions.

Performance Appraisals and Salary Administration

Performance appraisals are periodic meetings, usually held annually, between the employee and administrator or supervisor to discuss the employee's job performance. This is the administrator's opportunity to assess the employee's job performance within a specific period. During this period, the administrator should be observing how the employee carries out his job responsibilities. The administrator will be taking note of how the employee gets along with coworkers, his work ethic, promptness and ability to meet deadlines.

Discipline and counseling should take place on a regular basis. It is not a good idea to wait until the annual performance appraisal to address an employee's misconduct or poor performance. Corrective performance discussions can be scheduled at any time when it becomes necessary to advise the employee of poor performance and specify corrective action. The administrator should use this opportunity to outline a program for improved performance and give the employee a time line to show improvement. (Refer to *Disciplinary Action*, page 51.)

Employees are often very tense about a performance appraisal. The practice administrator should make the experience as positive as possible. Even if it is necessary to caution an employee about poor performance, it can be done in an encouraging manner. While it is important to point out marginal or poor performance, it is equally important to praise and encourage.

Preparing for the Performance Appraisal

When preparing for the performance appraisal, have all your facts in order. Pull out the employee's personnel folder and check for any Corrective Action Forms.

The following information will be useful:

- *Attendance records.* How many times has the employee been tardy? How many days has he been absent?

- *Compliments or complaints.* Anytime a patient comments about an employee, good or bad, it should be recorded in the personnel record.

- *Disciplinary actions or warning notices.*

- *The job description.* This is necessary to judge how well the employee is performing each task listed in the job description.

- *Performance goals.* In previous appraisals or counseling sessions, you should have set specific goals for improvement. Check to see how well the employee has completed these goals.

Performance appraisals, like all other employment decisions, are governed by state and federal labor laws and regulations. To avoid discrimination, administer appraisals fairly and consistently for all employees. Use the same, pre-printed form for every employee to assure that the same performance criteria will be used for every appraisal.

(See *Employee Performance Appraisal Form* — Exhibit 3-4.)

Laws and regulations governing performance appraisals are virtually the same as those governing the interviewing and hiring of employees.

- Focus on objective, job-related criteria.

- Concentrate on quantity and quality of work and completion of job-related goals.

- Avoid subjective criteria such as demeanor, bearing, manner, or social behavior.

- Rate good and bad performance.

- Provide a copy to the employee and keep a copy in the personnel record.

- Have the employee sign the performance appraisal. Explain that signing the form does not necessarily indicate agreement with management's finding. However, it does indicate that the employee was informed of the problems. *If the employee refuses to sign the form, indicate this in writing and sign the form.*

- Document any disciplinary action at the time it occurs. Management's motive in a poor performance discharge may be questioned if the poor performance was not documented at the time of the disciplinary action.

- *Do not avoid poor performance ratings for fear of discrimination charges.* Address performance issues for all employees on a consistent and timely basis.

- Clearly specify a final warning on the Performance Appraisal or Corrective Action Form.

- Avoid back-dating appraisals or unusually harsh treatment of the employee to force resignation.

- ***Be consistent.*** Inconsistency will reflect poorly on any legal proceedings that may arise.

- If poor performance is used to deny or delay a pay adjustment, document clearly and thoroughly.

- Do not make any discriminatory comments during the performance appraisal or on the appraisal form.

Twenty-Two Tips for Productive Performance Discussions

1. *Be Prepared.* Define work place policies and clarify performance standards to achieve a consensus among administrators and physician. Define and use performance rating definitions. Participate in team performance ratings where administrators or physician rates employee performance. Take some time to be thorough in preparing the performance appraisal form. Complete all parts of the form, including written comments to praise, critique, or clarify a rating. Careful preparation will promote a more meaningful performance discussion.

2. *Plan Your Discussion.* Carefully plan your discussion with the employee. Use the performance appraisal form as an outline to guide the discussion. Try to anticipate the employee's reaction to your performance ratings. Consider how you will respond to the employee's reaction. If you properly provided daily performance feedback during the rating period, there should be no surprises. Rather, the performance discussion will be a review of issues already discussed with the employee.

3. *Get Approvals.* Performance appraisals and any pay adjustments should be approved by the physician prior to discussion with the employee.

4. *Notify Employee.* Notify the employee in advance regarding the performance appraisal discussion. Many practices schedule performance appraisals to coincide with one's employment anniversary or some other designated day of the year. When you notify the employee in advance, you promote more open and positive communications. Advance notice lets the employee know that you are prepared to discuss performance and pay issues on a timely basis.

5. *Collect Work Samples.* Collect any facts, documents, reports, work samples, or other similar items that reflect the employee's job output. These samples will be useful to illustrate the employee's performance, promote objective evaluation of performance, and help to justify performance ratings. Use of work samples focuses discussion to specific job output issues. Be aware of the tendency to generalize overall performance based on a single "likeable" characteristic. Constructive suggestions on how to perform tasks more efficiently help to minimize emotional confrontations.

6. *Allow Adequate Time.* To have a meaningful discussion, be sure to allow adequate time to discuss job expectations and the employee's performance. As a general guide, performance discussions with employees in more complex jobs such as skilled, administrative, professional,

or management positions should be 30 minutes to an hour or more. The key factor is to allot sufficient time to discuss job requirements, rate the employee's performance, suggest ways to improve and to elicit employee response.

7. *Avoid Interruptions.* Pick an interview time and place where interruptions will be minimized or avoided. A private office, conference room, or an area away from the main flow of work are possible locations for performance appraisal discussions. It is disconcerting to have other employees walking by or coming into an office during a performance discussion. Telephone calls also disrupt the performance discussion. Make an effort to prevent or avoid these interruptions. Avoid performance discussions over lunch.

8. *Describe the Process.* By describing the purpose, process, and result of the performance appraisal discussion to the employee, you reduce the uncertainty and answer some of his or her questions. Secondly, it helps you to take charge of the discussion by defining what issues will be discussed.

9. *Be Friendly, Yet Businesslike.* The tone of the performance appraisal discussion should be friendly, positive and businesslike. Avoid joking or nervous laughter during the discussion. Try to encourage the employee to relax. If the employee has serious or continuing performance problems, your manner should be more firm to convey the seriousness of the employee's poor performance.

10. *Stay on Track.* Keep to the subject at hand. Do not let the discussion wander into unrelated areas. Thorough preparation will help you to discuss specific performance issues and minimize unrelated discussions.

11. *Follow the Appraisal Form.* One easy way to set a direction to the discussion is to follow the performance appraisal form. First, identify the performance factor, then the desired performance norm, and then your rating of the employee's performance. When you compare the results of the employee's work to the expected norm, issues can be discussed on a more objective basis. Avoid personal criticisms or insulting remarks.

12. *Praise Achievements.* Recognition and praise for achievements is an important part of the performance appraisal process. Giving credit, when due, helps the employee to know his or her efforts are recognized. Recognition is an effective motivator.

13. *Identify Deficiencies.* Poor performance must be clearly identified and marked on the performance appraisal form and discussed with the employee. Be direct. Give specific examples of performance problems and then identify the desired level of performance. The employee will assume that performance is satisfactory unless the problems are specifically identified.

14. *Sandwich Technique.* This technique can be helpful when discussing performance problems. First compliment the employee on an aspect of good performance, then identify a performance deficiency, and then follow up with another comment about good performance. Clearly, this technique softens the effect of discussing poor performance. Avoid overusing this technique. In cases of serious or repeated poor performance, be sure to describe the problem specifically and specify the desired performance.

15. *Maintain Professionalism.* The performance appraisal discussion should be constructive, not confrontational; pleasant and professional, not a contest of personalities; with an element of empathy rather than pitched emotion. Focus on job tasks, results and accomplishments. Personal attacks upon the individual are likely to arouse an argumentative response or result in barriers to communication.

16. *Offer Improvement Suggestions.* Offer specific suggestions on how to improve performance, particularly when identifying performance problems. Performance improvement is not likely to occur merely by identifying the employee's mistakes. However, performance improvement is more likely when the employee understands proper work techniques and expected performance goals.

17. *Set Performance Goals.* One key to improved performance is setting performance goals. By defining performance goals, the employee has a target to work toward. To be effective, goal-setting should include employee input. Goals should be achievable with some extra effort. Defined goals provide a ready basis to evaluate performance during the next rating period.

18. *Discuss Performance, Then Pay.* Performance appraisal and pay adjustment discussions may be together. It is best to discuss performance first, and then explain how the performance rating has influenced the pay adjustment. Some employers set these discussions for two separate meetings to maximize each issue.

19. *Don't Discredit the Practice.* Occasionally, an inexperienced administrator may promise a pay raise or tell the employee that a recommended pay raise was cut by management. When an administrator discredits the practice in this fashion, this action really reflects poorly on the administrator. Do not fall into this trap.

20. *Encourage Employee Comments.* A primary objective of the performance appraisal is communication between employees and administrators. Accordingly, encourage your employees to react to the performance ratings. The employee may agree, disagree, or offer reasons (sometimes excuses) for performance problems. Listen to and consider the employee's comments. Allow the employee to suggest ways the efficiency of his position might be improved.

21. *Discuss Employee Goals.* What does the employee want or need in the way of personal development or training? What are his future career goals? What additional responsibilities might be added to his current position, if any? Is there a possibility of upward mobility?

22. *Employee Signature.* Most performance appraisal forms have a space for an employee signature. At the conclusion of the performance appraisal discussion, ask the employee to sign the form. The employee's signature serves to acknowledge that the performance discussion occurred. Also, many performance appraisal forms have a space for employee comments. In the interest of constructive communication, invite the employee to make written comments.

Salary Administration

Discussing salary with an employee is a challenging responsibility for the administrator. There are many psychological factors surrounding the employee's perception about pay. A pay increase, or lack of increase, directly affects an employee's self esteem, morale and perception of his value to the practice.

Careful preparation for the discussion of pay issues is important to protect the employee's morale and to encourage him to strive to improve regardless of pay increases. The following tips will help you to have a successful meeting with your employees about pay.

- Make sure you know everything about the practice's philosophy about pay.
- Obtain approval or discuss the allowed percentage of increase with the physician prior to conducting salary reviews.
- Protect confidentiality. Do not discuss or compare one employee's salary or abilities with another.
- Discuss the relationship between pay and performance.
- Be specific in discussing any performance problems that deny, reduce or delay a pay adjustment.
- Respond honestly to any questions about pay without violating confidentiality guidelines.
- Take the responsibility to present pay issues to the employees in a way that emphasizes the positive aspects of employment.
- Discuss performance first, pay second.
- Explain how practice conditions, the economy and practice growth affect pay raises.
- Give the employee a statement of all his benefits, including insurance, vacation, sick pay and required government benefits.
- It is critical that you conduct reviews on or very near the date they are due. If the appraisal is delayed for an insignificant reason, it tells the employee you are not concerned about them or their performance.

Because of the ever-increasing cost of operating a medical practice, it is often necessary to explain to employees that finances prevent any pay increases.

Employees should always be made aware of the cost of operations in the practice. Solicit their help and ideas in keeping costs down. Let employees know what steps management has taken to reduce costs. If you have "kept the employees in the loop," they will not be surprised when you announce the news that there will be no raises this year. You may not have to make this announcement if you and the employees have made a concerted effort to save money in other areas.

Emphasize the need for teamwork, cooperation and continued effort by all employees to get through these tough times. Avoid making promises of future pay raises or commitments about job security. Such promises, if unfulfilled, will further erode morale. *Do not, under any circumstances, discredit or blame the physician for the lack of pay increases!*

Employee perception of pay is a factor in turnover, absences, morale and motivation. For these reasons, it is important to effectively communicate pay information.

(See *Salary Change Recommendation Form* — Exhibit 3-5.)

Disciplinary Action

Performance Problems

A performance problem is generally defined as *an action or inaction that causes work tasks to be performed poorly or in a manner that fails to meet expectations.* Errors in completion of reports or data, inability to complete tasks on time, and failure to meet standards for quality and quantity of work are all examples of poor performance.

The administrator should address performance problems as soon as they become apparent. Any employee can have a bad day or a bad week. However, if poor performance continues for more than a few days, a counseling session is in order.

In order to fairly judge if an employee is performing up to expectations, there must be guidelines for performance, such as a job description.

Thoroughly explain to the employee the areas of the poor performance. Outline specific instruction for how the performance should be improved. Give a definite time line for improvement. Set a specific date for another meeting to discuss progress. Above all, stick to your own time line and monitor progress daily.

Document all corrective action. Obtain the employee's signature on the Corrective Action Form and place a copy in the employee's personnel file.

Misconduct Problems

Misconduct is defined as *a violation of policy or published rules.* Common examples may include theft, insubordination, use of drugs or alcohol, or excessive absenteeism.

Refer to The Employee Handbook when addressing a misconduct incident with an employee. Disciplinary action for misconduct commonly takes the form of verbal warnings, written warnings, suspension without pay and ultimately discharge.

If the warning is verbal, record the date of the warning and a brief description of the infraction in the employee's personnel record. For example:

> *June 25, 1995. Maryann was warned about her absenteeism today. (Signature.)*

You may choose to give two verbal warnings before a written Corrective Action Form is completed. (See *Corrective Action Form* — Exhibit 3-6.) The disciplinary process should be described in The Employee Handbook and the guidelines followed exactly for every case of poor performance or misconduct.

Other corrective action tips:

- Investigate the incident.
- Verify facts, check records, get statements from "witnesses."
- Speak with the employee in private.
- Specify the nature of the misconduct and why it is inappropriate.

- Specify what corrective action must be taken.

- Specify what happens if the misconduct continues (for instance, suspension or termination).

The most important factor in dealing with disciplinary problems is to document the incident and assure that the documentation is factual and complete.

Termination

Employment related/work related lawsuits have skyrocketed during the last 20 years by more than 2,000 percent! This increase in litigation, combined with the fact that recruiting and training a new employee is expensive and time-consuming, prevents us from discharging unsuitable employees often enough or soon enough. When a great deal of money and effort is spent on employees that are not producing, the productive employees feel cheated.

Here are five steps to a legal termination process.

- ***Act on problems immediately.*** Employees most likely to sue are those who think they have been fired unjustly. Communicate with them about poor performance immediately and track their improvement, if any, through weekly or monthly sessions.

- ***Document thoroughly.*** Use written Corrective Action Forms and conduct regular performance appraisals. Be specific in describing an incidence of poor performance or misconduct. Make sure there is documentation of every session with an employee.

- ***Include the employee.*** Have the employees evaluate themselves. If problems are acknowledged, you are much closer to resolutions. If they are denied, you may have ammunition in court that the employee did not respond to constructive criticism.

- ***Act quickly.*** If the employee's performance does not improve after counseling, do not delay the decision. There is no **legal** reason why you must document disciplinary action but you must follow your practice's policy. Avoid claims of discrimination by having the documentation for the issue of termination.

- ***Be candid.*** Explain to the employee the reason for the termination. Have someone else present from the practice to witness and record the termination and the employee's responses.

- ***Prepare a Termination Checklist.*** Collect any keys or materials from the employee that belong to the practice. Have the final check ready. If the employee has insurance through the practice, explain the COBRA benefits. (See Chapter 2, *Employee Relations* for further information about COBRA. Also, see *Termination Employee Checklist —* Exhibit 3-7.)

- ***Reassure other employees.*** When an employee is terminated, it may affect the morale of the other employees. They may feel like they will be next. Take the time to explain what happened and explain that you have no plans to fire anyone else.

After a termination is complete, do a "post-mortem." Review all your data on the employee. What was unacceptable about the employee? How could the termination have been prevented? A firing experience may provide an opportunity to evaluate your management skills. A thorough analysis of the termination will force you to change your focus from managing things to leading people.

The Employee Handbook

The Employee Handbook may be one of the most useful tools in your practice. It provides the employee with a written guide to practice policy and benefits. It also helps the manager by furnishing a reference for fair and impartial administration of policies and benefits. With practice policies, work rules, and benefits in writing, many complaints and misunderstandings can be dealt with quickly and easily. Written policies reduce the risk of a lawsuit being brought by a disgruntled employee who feels unfairly treated or unjustly discharged.

One word of caution is to avoid the handbook serving as an employment contract by prominently placing an "employment at-will" disclaimer in the book.

Writing an employee handbook is a significant undertaking. Begin by considering what you want your staff to understand. A well-written handbook will answer these questions:

- What is expected of the employee and the employer?

- What are the policies on wages, working conditions, and benefits?

- What services does your practice provide to patients?

Use the handbook to express the following:

- The philosophy of the physician and the mission of the practice.

- A sense of security to employees a sense of being a part of something.

- What is expected of the employee.

- What is provided by the employer.

- How to get help with problems and information on benefits.

The administrator gains from preparing an employee handbook by reexamining practice policies and the level of understanding between managers and employees. Allow employees to participate in the process to attain a better level of communication. The handbook can set the framework for successful relationships between the employer and employees by identifying conditions of employment, what employers need to know to satisfy those conditions, and what assistance the practice will provide in meeting those conditions.

Make your book attractive and easy to use. Select a size that is neither too large nor too small. Typical sizes are 3 1/2" x 6 1/2" or 5" x 7". Loose leaf-binders allow for replacement of pages when policies or benefits change. Policy statements in handbooks should be general enough that they do not require frequent changes.

For ease in reading, follow these pointers:

- Limit the use of words with three or more syllables.

- Keep each sentence 20 words or less.

- Limit discussion of a subject to one page.

- Use drawings, charts, and cartoons where applicable.

- Leave at least one quarter of each page blank.

- Limit the number of pages (convey a simple message).

Choose a writing style and be consistent throughout. Use "you" and "your" if you wish to be personal. Or, approach policies in a general way by using an impersonal style. Another effective approach is to ask a question in the heading and then answer the question in the discussion below the heading.

Write clearly and to the point. Use sex-neutral terminology. Avoid gender-biased pronouns and expressions wherever possible. If writing is not your talent, get outside help with composition, grammar or style.

Include in the handbook what employees need to know to get along on the job. Working hours, dress codes and standards, break periods, paydays, absences, safety, and general information about the working environment should be addressed. The handbook should also describe what the practice offers in benefits and special services, such as vacations, leaves, medical benefits, jury duty, holidays, educational assistance, and insurance. Typically, the handbook also contains a welcome message, a short history of the practice, and a "disclaimer" statement. Arrange the contents by sections, such as (1) welcome and introduction, (2) employment policies, (3) benefits provided, and (4) employee responsibility including safety and discipline procedures. Use of a table of contents is helpful.

Handbooks vary due to individual needs and circumstances. The following sample table of contents can be used as a checklist for deciding what to include in the handbook.

- **Welcome Letter and Introduction**
    - Letter of Appreciation to Current Employees
    - Letter of Welcome to New Employees
    - Purpose of Handbook
    - Background of Practice
    - Organization Chart
    - Physician(s) Biographical Information, etc.
    - Equal Employment Opportunity Statement
    - Suggestion and Complaint Procedures

- **Employment Policies and Procedures**
    - Nature of Employment
    - Probationary Period
    - Employee Relations
    - Supervisor's Responsibilities
    - Employee's Role and Responsibilities
    - Work Schedules
    - Rest and Meal Periods
    - Overtime Policy
    - Attendance and Punctuality
    - Time Cards/Records
    - Personnel Records

- Payday
- Payroll Deductions
- Performance and Salary Reviews
- Resignation/Termination
- Telephone Use

■ **Benefits**
- Holidays
- Vacations
- Hospital and Medical Insurance
- Life Insurance
- Pension and Profit-Sharing
- Training
- Educational Assistance Program
- Service Awards
- Workers' Compensation
- Sick Leave
- Disability Leave
- Personal Leave
- Bereavement Leave
- Jury Duty
- Witness Duty

■ **Safety**
- Safety Rules
- Emergency Procedures
- Personal Protective Equipment
- Reporting Accidents

■ **Employee Conduct and Disciplinary Action**
- Standards of Conduct
- Confidentiality Policy
- Smoking Policy
- Drug, Alcohol, and Substance Abuse Policy
- Sexual and Other Forms of Impermissible Harassment
- Security Inspections
- Solicitation
- Personal Appearance Standards
- Dress Codes
- Corrective Discipline Procedures

■ **Summary and Acknowledgement**
- Disclaimer Statement

CHAPTER 4

Financial Management

Financial patterns in the medical practice are changing in the nineties. Reimbursements are reduced by government cut-backs in medical programs and the insurgence of managed care. Smart medical practice administrators today are planning long term, sustainable approaches to reducing costs and maximizing revenues.

Controlling costs only when business is bad is a "prescription for failure." A successful approach to saving is made up of incremental steps — a series of cost control measures that when strung together, lead to a leaner, more profitable practice.

This chapter provides you with some step-by-step methods to improve the financial performance of your practice. You will learn ways to maximize reimbursement and some simple, yet effective, cost cutting measures.

The Operating Budget

The operating budget is based on an annual average of operating expenses of the medical practice. You will be able to plan the spending requirements as they directly relate to the earnings of the practice. The budget will allow for preplanning ability to curb needless spending and unplanned purchasing.

The importance of an operating budget cannot be over-stressed. The basic concept is to:

- *Review* historical collections and spending, and

- *Plan* how much can be spent. The goal is to attain an *acceptable* level of income.

Your financial success depends on your knowledge and understanding of the complete financial workings of the practice. This includes knowing the cost of each service you deliver and the average cost of seeing a patient in the practice.

Do not be discouraged about the budgeting process. While you may perceive it as too complicated or time consuming, the method which follows is a simple process. It is fun, fascinating, and enlightening.

Benchmarking

One way to budget is to look at benchmarks for your specialty and strive for those averages. However, it is best to budget what you will spend to provide your net profit. Using this method, you will compare your expenses to those of other practices in your specialty nationwide. You will discover which areas you need to work on to reduce costs and some tips for reducing these costs.

To begin, gather the following documents:

- Your most recent year-end financial statement or the last six months report annualized.

- A copy of the *Practice Management Statistics* form (Exhibit 4-1). This form should be used at quarterly intervals so that you can see peaks and valleys in your practice operation's expenses and earnings.

- The *Major Expenses by Specialty* table (Exhibit 4-2, page 60, Table 1), shows the national averages for major expenditures in each specialty. If you have information from another source that is specific to your region, use those benchmarks. These statistics are provided annually by a number of sources. This data in this table is from the *Medical Group Management Association*.

Step 1 – Calculate your total expense-to-earning percentage. Divide total expenses by total collections. Check the national average to see where you stand.

Step 2 – Calculate the percentage of <u>collections minus refunds</u> for each of your practice's major expenditures. (Your CPA may have already provided this information on the financial statement.)

For example:

If your gross collections are $450,000 and your salary and wage expense (excluding physician salaries) is $80,000, your personnel costs are about 18 percent of your collections. Notice on the following chart that the national average is 17–24 percent for staff salaries. (You can perform these calculations on an electronic spread sheet if you have the appropriate computer software.)

Once you have calculated all the expenditure percentages, enter them on the *Practice Management Statistics Form*. Then place the national averages for your specialty on the form. Target the areas that exceed the national average.

TIP: Remember, benchmarks are only averages. Do you want your practice to be "just average"?

While "benchmarking" is a helpful tool, it only provides you with information about the average practice. The national statistics do not account for the various ancillary services provided by some practices which have a significant impact on revenue production.

National statistics, specific to your specialty, can be obtained through the *Medical Group Management Association* and through other sources.

Personnel Costs

The physician's philosophy, practice style, and the number of ancillary services you provide play a part in staffing levels. Find your specialty in the Staffing Ratios by Specialty table. Determine what your staff-to-physician ratio should be.

Staffing Ratios by Specialty

Family Practice	3.5 - 6.0
Internal Medicine	3.3 - 3.5
OB/GYN	3.2 - 4.3
Pediatrics	3.5 - 4.0
Otolaryngology	4.5 - 5.0
Cardiology	3.5 - 4.5
Neurology	3.6 - 4.0
Ophthalmology	5.2 - 6.4
General Surgery	2.5 - 3.0
Urology	3.5 - 3.8
Orthopedics	4.0 - 5.3
Gastroenterology	3.5 - 6.0
Psychiatry	1.8 - 2.2
Neurosurgery	3.3 - 4.5

Source: *Practice Support Resources, Inc.*

If your staff-to-physician ratio is in line and your percentage of expenditures is average, look for other areas to cut costs.

- If the ratio is right but the costs are too high, you may have long-term employees that have received pay raises every year. Or, competition for good people in your area may be high and higher salaries must be paid in order to compete. In either case, your options may be limited to "freezing" raises and finding innovative ways to reward employees. (See Chapter 2, *Salary Administration* for ideas.)

- If the ratio is right but your salary costs are 5–10 percent below the average, you may have several new employees at starting range, or there may be less competition for employees in your area. Evaluate your turnover rate. Are your salaries competitive? If your staff is underpaid, consider giving a small raise and see how efficiency picks up. In order to provide quality patient care, a practice needs quality as well as qualified personnel. It pays to invest wisely in your staff.

- Are staff expenditures too high and is your staff-to-physician ratio higher than the average? You may have some room for cost reduction. How is the efficiency in your practice? If efficiency is good but ratios are too high, you may want to keep all the employees but consider cutting back on hours. Do you have an employee with young children who would like to come in later or leave in time to be home with the children after school? You may reduce your expenses while making a staff member happy at the same time. Chances are there will be no decline in efficiency. Be innovative!

- If staff ratios and expenses are high yet work is left undone, you may have an efficiency problem. Take a close look at each employee, their job description, and how well they do their job. Commit to do what needs to be done. Make your employees accountable for efficiency and productivity. The survival of the practice may be at stake!

Major Expenses by Specialty

The chart/grid, shown as Table 1, provides 1995 data that will allow the practice to compare its expenses to other practices in the same specialty. The information is based on *national averages* and are intended for use only as a guideline. The physician's practice philosophy and the complexity of the practice may alter these averages for your specific practice.

Major Expenses by Specialty   Table 1

Expense Category	Cardiology	Family Medicine	GASTRO	Internal Medicine	OB/GYN	Opthal.	ENT	Pediatrics	Surgery General	Surgery Orthopedic
Personnel Salaries	17.41%	24.08%	15.79%	21.12%	17.78%	21.04%	18.45%	22.85%	14.30%	16.59%
Personnel Benefits	4.49%	5.32%	4.31%	5.11%	5.09%	4.80%	4.13%	4.78%	3.67%	4.72%
Rent	4.23%	6.79%	4.63%	6.16%	5.49%	7.18%	6.24%	6.18%	5.47%	5.44%
Lab	0.65%	3.26%	*	4.82%	2.80%	*	*	1.36%	*	0.11%
Medical Supplies	0.88%	3.36%	1.11%	2.08%	2.56%	1.71%	1.87%	7.46%	0.79%	2.07%
Administrative Supplies	1.52%	2.08%	*	1.65%	1.57%	1.74%	2.61%	1.58%	1.20%	1.62%
Malpractice1.40%	1.85%	1.53%	1.38%	5.03%	1.11%	1.22%	1.37%	4.12%	3.02%	
Legal and Accounting	0.55%	0.46%	0.60%	0.47%	0.65%	0.74%	0.60%	0.51%	0.76%	0.66%
Promotions/Marketing	0.43%	0.35%	*	0.29%	0.52%	1.47%	0.72%	0.39%	0.39%	0.57%
Operating Overhead	**42.93%**	**56.34%**	**40.43%**	**53.64%**	**48.70%**	**54.49%**	**45.78%**	**54.18%**	**38.66%**	**42.46%**

Used by Permission from Medical Group Management Association

Medical and Administrative Expenses

- **Purchasing.** Supply cost is generally the second largest expense in a medical practice and an area where there is almost always room for improvement. After comparing your costs to the national averages, consider these tips for cost reduction.

  Institute an employee suggestion box for cost-cutting ideas. Give a "prize" each month for the best recommendation that actually saves the practice money. Keep the staff involved by letting them decide which suggestion is best.

  Take advantage of free items. Pens, pencils, note pads and even personalized prescription pads are provided by almost every pharmaceutical sales representative and other vendors.

  Eliminate frills such as buying four types of pens to suit various employees.

  Ask your staff to concentrate on saving money in supplies for a specific period. If expenses are measurably reduced, reward them with a special treat such as lunch or a small bonus.

  Purchase at the best possible price.
  - Ask medical supply vendors to give you the "hospital" price.
  - Consider ordering generic goods rather than name brand items.
  - Order in bulk non-sterile, loose, multi-packed dry goods.
  - Ask about drop shipments.
  - Buy at year end.
  - Conduct price comparisons every six months. List the items most often used and circulate this list to the vendors of choice. Include the size and quantity of each.
  - Identify suppliers who provide the best quality for the money (local manufacturers, discount houses, catalog purchasing).

- **Outsourcing.** As medical practices are increasingly burdened with administrative paperwork, outsourcing offers a popular alternative to adding personnel. The decision to outsource may reduce administrative headaches and save money in the process.

  Outsourcing is not really new. Many practices outsource accounting services.

  - **Billing and Collections.**   Many practices hire an outside agency to provide these services on a percentage basis. When considering agencies, for better collection results, select one that bases its cost on collections rather than charges.

    If you are considering changing or upgrading your computer system to accommodate billing functions, first investigate the possibility of outsourcing the billing and collection functions. The fees for these services are usually 5–10 percent of total collections. The cost of doing this in-house will most likely exceed 10 percent in addition to the cost of a new or upgraded computer system.

    When outsourcing, also choose a billing and collections service that will track managed care billings and payments by each individual plan.

– *Payroll.* The payroll function is easily outsourced to companies that specialize in automated payroll processing. Because of volume and sophisticated computer systems, they provide these services at a fraction of the cost of handling the payroll and the associated tax functions in-house. (See page 67 for further discussion on Payroll Administration.)

– *Employee Staffing.* A newer trend in outsourcing is employee leasing. The office setting and daily operations remain the same, except the employees are on another company's payroll. The leasing company pays for the employees' salary and benefits, then bills the physician's practice. The physician still has hiring and firing authority and determines the salary of the staff member.

Employee leasing provides a cost saving in fringe benefits. By leasing, you may be able to afford benefits for your employees that previously have been too costly. By having more employees to pool, leasing companies are able to obtain lower rates than small businesses.

■ *Vendor Relations.* Establish relationships with reliable, service-oriented vendors who offer good products at fair prices. Open accounts with businesses who will work with you on cost reductions for bulk purchases and drop shipments. Consider buying items in a one-year or six-month supply; have necessary quantities dropped to you at specific time intervals.

Order bulk purchases at year-end if possible. Sales representatives will offer the best prices at that time in an attempt to reach year-end sales quotas. Be familiar with price breaks for regularly used items so that you can purchase in quantities that provide discounts.

Create vendor files by company name and file all invoices and statements in chronological order. File the folders in alphabetical order.

Keep stock closets locked and off limits to vendors. Most sales representatives are honest. However, occasionally a sales rep will say you are short on particular items and order more, even those you seldom use.

Consider purchasing office supplies in person from a "discount" office supply store rather than ordering from a vendor who delivers. To cover the cost of delivery, some local office supply businesses may charge more for supplies.

Having a charge card eliminates the need for check approval and signature. *Place strict controls on the use of this charge card and require that accurate records and receipts be kept on all purchases.*

■ *Inventory Control.* Every office should have an inventory control system for all purchases from office supplies to laboratory and X-ray supplies. A good inventory system not only increases efficiency but controls costs. Establish a supply inventory control system to:

– Prevent ordering supplies already on hand.

– Prevent over-ordering.

– Reduce high volume of shelved goods.

Most practices have some supplies that have been around for years that are seldom used. Know what you use, how much you use, and order only when supplies are needed. Have an office supply "round-up" at east twice a year. Clean out every desk and every closet, gathering pens/pencils, paper clips, pads, etc. Use the supplies you have on hand and do not order unnecessarily.

Try this simple Order Point System to control the amount of inventory on hand, to minimize overstocking, and to prevent shortages. To use this system, determine the following:

1. The quantity of material or inventory item used in a 30-day period.

2. The time between order and receipt of goods.

3. The quantity of item needed during the period of time required in #2.

4. The level of buffer stock necessary in the event of an interruption of supply.

Example:
Your office uses 100 5cc syringes per month.
It takes 12 days from the date of order to the date of delivery.
Your office uses about 50 syringes in 12 days.
You should have a buffer stock of 100 syringes in case of back order.
You should order when your inventory reaches 150 syringes.
If 5cc syringes come 100 to a box, you should tag the next to last box with a sticker that says, Order Now.
You will use 50 syringes before your order is delivered, and you will have a safety stock of at least 100 syringes when your new order arrives.

- *Ordering Logs.* Use order logs to track the date an order was placed for supplies, the quantity, and the cost quotes for each item.
    - Cross-check packing slips with order log entries. Cross-check monthly statements with packing slips.
    - Note in the log when a generic form of a product was ordered.

- *Bartering.* Consider exchanging or trading one service for another. Trade a complete physical exam for carpet cleaning or painting. It may save you money toprovide a procedure such as a physician exam to one of your patients in exchange for carpet cleaning service, painting, etc. It is important to document what you trade and the value of each service.

    Write to The International Reciprocal Trade Association at 9513 Beach Mill Road, Great Falls, VA 22066 for information about a barter group in your area.

- *Occupancy Expense.* There may not be much you can do about your rent expenses unless you are at the end of a lease period and office space is abundant. As your renewal date approaches, negotiate for a lower rental fee, or at least strive for no escalation.

    Save money on utilities. Heating and cooling bills can be reduced by using an electronic thermostat that automatically adjusts the temperature at a preset time. Raise or lower your settings according to the seasonal changes. Insulate windows to keep the controlled air inside. Insulate the hot water heater. Use the same cost-saving ideas you would use in your home.

- ***Malpractice Insurance.*** Research and negotiate malpractice policies every year. While this is time consuming, it may save you money. As you see rate variances among insurance carriers, be sure to compare equivalent coverage.

- ***Legal and Accounting Fees.*** If you pay an outside accountant for monthly financial statements, you may be spending several thousand dollars each year in accounting fees. Consider having statements prepared by the accountant quarterly rather than monthly. If you are financially inclined, prepare monthly statements in-house. Purchase an accounting software package for your computer that will allow you to prepare financial statements.

- ***Service Contracts.*** Examine your service contracts to see if they are needed and worth the cost. Contracts on highly reliable equipment are a waste of money. Fax machines, telephones, personal computers, calculators, and high quality laser printers seldom malfunction. Often, service contracts cost more than repair or replacement of the equipment. Avoid long-term service contracts or those that renew automatically. If you have paid up contracts, take advantage of everything you are due, such as routine maintenance and cleaning.

- ***Petty Cash.*** Establish a petty cash fund (usually about $50.00) to pay incidental expenses. Begin by drawing and cashing a check. Place the cash with a designated employee who is authorized to disburse the fund according to guidelines and restrictions for the amount and purpose. When a disbursement is made, the details are recorded by the designated employee on a receipt form. The signature of the payee is obtained, and the completed form is initialed. When the petty cash fund is reduced to a predetermined amount, the fund is replenished to the original amount. (See *Petty Cash Fund* — Exhibit 4-1.)

Establish a few ground rules for your Petty Cash Fund.

- The Petty Cash Fund is not to be used for cashing personal checks.
- Every disbursement must have a receipt to back it up.
- Do not use the Petty Cash fund to make change.
- Use a disbursements form to track petty cash spending.
- Designate one person in charge of petty cash.
- Maintain funds and receipts in a locked box.
- Do not allow borrowing from the Petty Cash fund.

Tracking Revenues

Successful revenue management requires you to have in-depth knowledge of the source of revenues. If the practice specialty is primary care, the majority of your revenues are from patient visits. In a surgical specialty, funds are generated primarily from hospital surgeries.

It is important to take one step further and discover what percentage each payor contributes to your revenues. This information may be available on a report generated by your computer software called Revenue by Financial Classification. This report should be as finite as possible. Sort your information by each major managed care contract and by Medicare and Medicaid. Know how much each managed care contract contributes to your revenues to see how much revenue is at risk if you lose the contract.

(For further information on Managed Care Contracting, refer to the **PRACTICE SUCCESS!**© Series topic entitled *Managing Managed Care in the Medical Practice* published by Coker Publishing, LLC.)

Determining Profitability

Look at each service you deliver from an expense standpoint. Review lab and x-ray costs compared to collections from these areas. Also factor in personnel costs.

Calculate the average cost for seeing a patient to enable you to determine the profitability of each capitated contract. Unless you know how much it costs to treat a patient, you cannot successfully negotiate a capitated fee. Use the form on page 66, *Patient Cost Analysis*, to determine your cost per patient.

Remember, expenses fall into two categories: *fixed and variable.* For this calculation, you are only concerned with variable expenses.

Revenue and Expense

Fixed Expenses: (remain the same regardless of patient volume)

- Rent
- Equipment Leases
- Salary and Benefits
- Utilities
- Dues and Subscriptions
- Taxes

Variable Expenses: (vary with patient volume)

- Medical Supplies
- Office Supplies
- Lab Fees
- Transcription Service
- X-ray Supplies

Patient Cost Analysis

1. Total number of patients seen for prior 12 months .... _______________

2. Total of all expenses for prior 12 months .... _______________

3. Subtract from line 2 all fixed expenses (rent, salaries
    and benefits, insurance, utilities) .... _______________

4. Total patient expenses for prior 12 months .... _______________

5. Total receipts for prior 12 months .... _______________

6. Divide line 5 by line 1 to get gross revenue per patient .... _______________

7. Divide line 4 by line 1 to get cost per patient .... _______________

8. Subtract line 7 from line 6 to get revenue per patient .... _______________

Computerized information systems provide a tremendous amount of financial information about the practice. While this information is valuable, it is often difficult to extrapolate specific information the physician and administrator need on a monthly basis. The use of a summary report will provide this vital information in a "quick read" fashion. The reports should be kept in a three-ring binder for easy reference and comparison.

Two such summary reports are shown as Exhibits 1 and 4-4.

Accounts Payable Management

Definition: Accounts payable — A liability representing an amount owed to a creditor, usually arising from purchase of merchandise or materials and supplies, not necessarily due or past due. Normally, a current liability, arising from the day-to-day operation of the business.

A primary function of the administrator is accounts payable management. Responsibilities include purchasing and paying bills.

Purchasing

Begin developing an organized purchasing system by centralizing the process. Assign one person to be responsible for ordering supplies. In a large practice, office supplies may be ordered by the practice administrator and medical supplies ordered by a nurse manager. This eliminates duplication of orders, adds objectivity, and prevents having sales representatives talking to various staff members. The employee in charge of purchasing becomes familiar with supplies and prices offered by the vendors so that he or she can shop around for the best bargain.

While the use of formal purchase order forms is generally reserved for large practices, some type of purchase request form, order log, or "want list" should be used for ordering supplies. Track the date items were ordered, the date the order was placed, the quantity, and the price quotes for every item. When ordering a generic brand of drug, make a notation on the log. If the supplier ships a higher priced "brand" name when a generic has been ordered, you will have documentation to support your request.

Here are tips for purchasing:

- Develop a bulk ordering system controlled by a 30-day or quarterly time table.

- Percentage discounts are generated when purchase amounts exceed a predetermined level.

- Create an inventory listing of all supplies and equipment found on the premises.

- Create "vendor files" by company name and file invoices and statements in chronological order. File the folders in alphabetical order.

- Every six months, check the prices you pay for common items and compare vendor pricing to ensure that you are getting the best quality and price. Ask for competitive bids from three different vendors on supply items.

- The employee responsible for placing orders should be required to check the current stock to prevent over-ordering or running short.

- Control rush orders. Crisis ordering can increase the price as much as 25 percent.

- Communicate with the vendor when commitments are not met. There is no excuse for poor service.

Paying Bills

Never pay bills directly from a vendor's statement. Rather, pay from an invoice.

To avoid duplicate payment or payment for goods not received, tight controls must be maintained on invoices and packing slips. The person using the supply should be required to validate the item when received. Notations should be made on the packing slip of any discrepancies or problems with the supplies. Then the packing slip should be submitted to the person responsible for paying the bill. The practice administrator or bookkeeper will then compare the packing slip to the invoice before payment is made to ensure that all items have been received and are in good condition.

Following are tips for paying bills:

- Pay accounts by invoice, not statements. Compare invoices to packing slips and invoices to statements.

- Pay bills once a month unless a discount is given for payment in less than 30 days. Generally, 3–15 percent discounts are given on the total statement amount.

Payroll

Following is an overview of responsibilities for payroll administration in a medical practice.

- Have employees complete a new IRS Form W-2 at the beginning of each calendar year.

- Obtain the most current Internal Revenue Service information and guidelines for preparing deductions to ensure the correct amounts are withheld from each employee's earnings.

- Obtain the most current information from your state government for withholding requirements.

- Become familiar with the IRS and state revenue service forms for reporting staff salaries; follow the guidelines for filing.

- Treat all payroll information with confidentiality. Keep records in a secure place.

- Most important, seek advice from your accountant on proper reporting guidelines of employee earning information.

Accounts Receivable Management

Definition: Accounts receivable — a claim against a debtor usually arising from sales or services rendered, not necessarily due or past due. Normally, a current asset, and arising from the normal course of business.

Practice profitability is a direct product of successful revenue management. Once the service is rendered to the patient and a charge is added to your accounts receivable, the collection process should begin immediately. This section addresses the billing process and introduces techniques for control and collection of the part of the accounts receivable that will be paid by the patient.

Patient Policy Education

Patients should always be informed of the practice's financial payment policy when they call for their initial appointment. But do not let phone calls be the last mention of the practice's financial policy.

Have a written financial policy that is included in the practice brochure, on the New Patient Information Form, and on signs in the reception area. Reinforce the financial policy throughout a patient's relationship with the practice by including bill stuffers with statements. This is an easy, low-cost way to remind patients of their payment responsibilities. (More on *The Written Financial Payment* Policy follows.)

TIP: REMEMBER — No matter how well you educate your patients, your financial payment policy will only work if you follow through with it!

Collecting at the Time of Service

Patients should have a clear understanding of the practice's collection expectations.

An office sign indicating PAYMENT IS EXPECTED AT THE TIME OF SERVICE is an acceptable way of alerting patients that you expect payment for services before they leave the office.

It is often challenging to collect from patients while maintaining their goodwill. Having the right person and personality assigned to this responsibility can greatly enhance the collection process. For best results, make sure your collections clerk has a firm but pleasant manner, is well-trained in collection protocol, and is mature and experienced in dealing face-to-face with the public.

TIP: The challenge is to collect accounts due while maintaining the patient's good will.

When collecting from patients at the time of an office visit, there is one general rule that is basic, universal, and more effective than any other alternative —*Ask for the money.*

Remember, cash-flow is the very lifeblood of the practice. As soon as a patient leaves the office without paying, you begin to lose money. Most patients do not object to being asked to pay at the time of service. Often, it is *how* they are asked that is objectionable.

The Written Financial Payment Policy

Adopt a written financial payment policy for your practice. This policy should be part of the *Welcome to the Practice* information mailed to each new patient before the initial visit or presented at the time of the first visit to the office.

Tailor the financial policy to your specific practice and specialty. Outline for the patient how your office personnel handles patient billing, insurance filing and payment plans.

The financial policy works best when it is presented to the new patient as a separate form. Ask for the patient's signature on the form and make it part of the medical record. Consider these pointers for communicating your financial policy.

- Use it a simple, one-page form.
- Avoid any legal terminology.
- Define parameters for filing insurance, e.g., for services over $100.00, or for surgical or hospital services.
- Be flexible.

Patient Billing

Patient statements should be:

- Consistent.
- Clear.
- Concise.
- Easy to understand (no abbreviations).
- Professional in appearance.
- An accurate reflection of all charges and payments.
- Mailed at the same time each month (with a return envelope enclosed).

The Written Collection Policy

The day-to-day collection process is often neglected in the medical practice, primarily due to the lack of a collection routine or policy. Provision of a written collection policy and procedure enables the practice personnel to successfully handle collection issues.

The purpose of a written collection policy and procedure is to:

- Educate staff members to protocol.
- Educate patients to comply with established practice collection policies.
- Maintain revenue/income balance.

- Control the accounts receivable balance (at least 90 percent of A/R should be aged 30 days or less).

- Augment the collection ratio.

- Manage cycle billing systems.

- Track and define revenue from third party payer sources.

Keys to Successful Collecting

The success of any collection program depends on the persistence and commitment of the employees responsible. The collection process should be assigned to one employee as his or her primary responsibility. Key points to remember are:

- Telephone contacts are more effective than writing a letter.

- Delinquent accounts of 120 days from the date of service should be turned over to a collection agency.

- Strict adherence to the collection process assures the practice will maintain a healthy cash flow.

Collections

Collection procedures determine the profitability of the practice. There are two ways to measure the success of the collection system:

1. The collection ratio.

2. The accounts receivable balance.

Imbalance in collections, like lack of practice growth, throws off the overhead ratio, since overhead is directly related to the volume of work that is done.

The collection ratio is total collections divided by total charges less adjustments.
(Total collections ÷ total charges – adjustments = collection ratio.)

Collection Ratio

Monthly

Total Charges....................................$50,000

Total Receipts $30,000

Accounts Receivable........................$20,000

Total Receipts $30,000

Divided by Total Charges.................$50,000

Equals: 60%

Terminating the Physician-Patient Relationship

There may be occasions when it is necessary to terminate the physician-patient relationship. This usually occurs when the patient's account is turned over for collection or when the patient fails to follow a prescribed course of treatment.

A physician cannot refuse to give a patient an appointment because the patient has not paid the bill without first terminating the physician-patient relationship. The physician cannot refuse to release the patient's medical records because the bill has not been paid.

The amount of time that you are required to give a patient to seek health care elsewhere varies in each state. You are advised to contact your local medical society or attorney for an opinion about your area. This termination process protects you from having to see the patient who has not paid and gives you additional legal protection if the patient fails to follow your suggested treatment plan. (See Chapter 7, *Risk Management in the Medical Office* for sample letters of termination.)

Fees

Just as there is a close relationship between collections and a satisfactory flow of patients — with both factors related to the overhead of the practice — so it is with the assignment of fees.

The amount of productive time the doctor spends in his or her practice must produce sufficient income to permit the payment of overhead and achievement of an equitable and net income that is acceptable. To achieve this objective, the fees for a particular service are based directly on the amount of productive time that the physician devotes to rendering that service.

If the fees for performing a variety of services are set on the basis of a certain return per hour spent in their performance, then when the physician is working to capacity (satisfactorily busy, but not overloaded), his or her time will produce the necessary income to compensate satisfactorily.

If the relationship between fees for various services is not in balance, there will be peaks and valleys in the physician's dollar production.

In today's constantly changing reimbursement environment, relevant and timely information is essential for making informed decisions for the practice. The administrator and physician should know the ten procedures that have the greatest profit margin in the practice. Similarly, it is important to know the ten procedures that have the least profit margin.

To help physicians attain this data, computerized procedure analysis systems have been developed. Normally, cost procedure analysis is a combination of a computer software analysis combined with professional consultative evaluations. Such customized evaluations can reveal extensive and pertinent information specific to the practice.

Current principles of cost accounting, such as standard costing and contribution margin analysis, are applied to the procedure mix.

As a result of the information generated by the analysis, decisions can be made that affect various situations. These considerations may range from managed care contracting to changing reimbursement strategies. Potentially, a cost procedure analysis enables the practice to increase net collections, adjust fee levels, track profitability, discover coding anomalies, forecast the impact of capitation, and obtain valuable information for assessment of the operations of the practice.

In some practices, a customized cost procedures analysis is beyond the practice administrator's responsibilities. If needed, these services can be outsourced to a consulting firm with capabilities of completing the report. The exhibit below is an example of the outcome of a Cost Procedure Analysis for a specific CPT code.

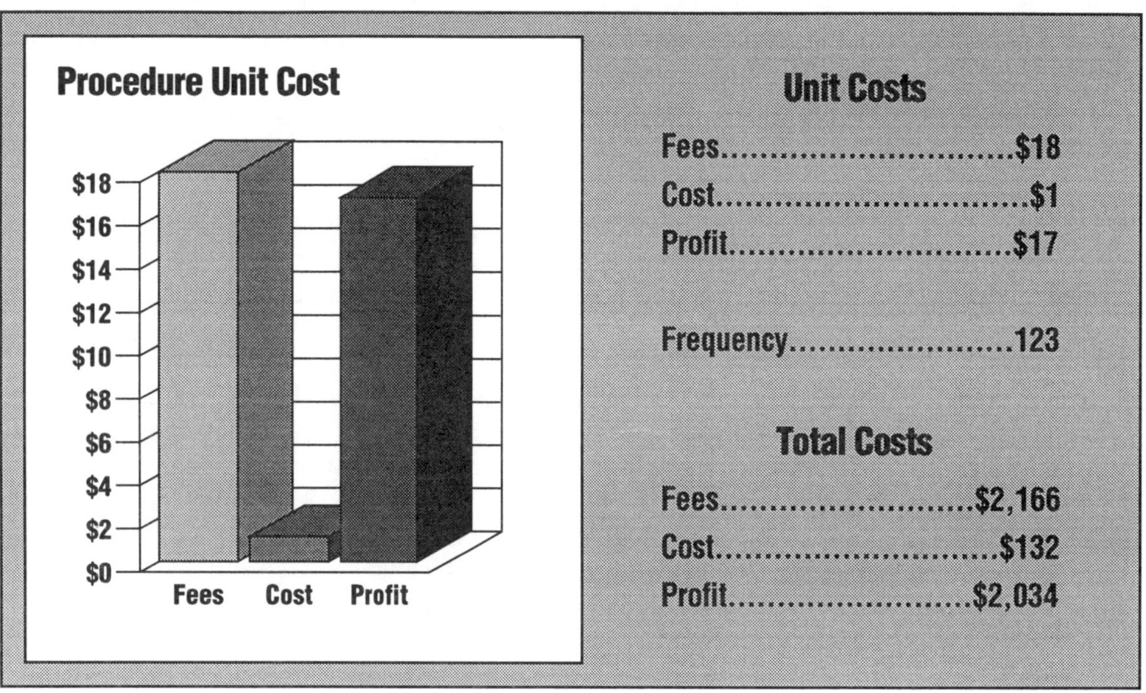

CHAPTER 5

Operations Management

Practice Policies and Procedures

In Chapter 3 we stressed the importance of The Employee Handbook to outline personnel policies. Equally important to the operation of the practice are business and administrative policies. This chapter will help you establish a policies and procedures manual to serve as an instruction guide for all employees.

A well-prepared, up-to-date policies and procedures manual is a definite time-saver for the administrator. Use it as an orientation and training guide as well as a reference to any employee that has a question about practice operations.

To begin preparing a policies and procedures manual, ask each employee to outline the steps they follow to perform each of their daily duties. From these outlines the administrator can write a policy for each task or procedure.

Procedure Manual

Procedure manuals used for instruction and establishing protocols should be written with greater detail and bound separately from the employee handbook. A medical practice should establish policy and protocol addressing OSHA, CLIA, and other government-regulated topics. Also included in the procedure manual are various operational protocols. Keep in mind the following points when writing procedures.

- Instructions should be straightforward and easy to understand.

- Procedures must be practical and easy to follow.

- Each policy should contain an effective date and revision date.

- Procedures should be updated regularly; copy of revised policies should be retained for 10 years.

- The manual should address issues confronted in the daily operation of the practice.

The contents should include written instructions on handling the following operational issues of the practice:

- **Office policies, including:**
  - Medical records
  - Release of information
  - Documentation

- Telephone advice
- Telephone technique
- Follow-up on abnormal lab results
- Scheduling
- Billing/collections
- Referrals/consults
- Discharging patients
- Patient education/instructions
- Patient relations
- Patient Confidentiality

- **Clinical procedures, including:**
  - Treatment protocols
  - Lab tests
  - X-ray

- **Emergencies and Safety, including:**
  - Emergency number (911, poison control, police, fire, etc.)
  - Staff members' responsibilities
  - First Aid training
  - CPR training

- **General Health and Safety, including:**
  - Bloodborne Pathogens Exposure Control Plan
  - OSHA Recordkeeping and Posting Requirements
  - OSHA Personal Protective Equipment Standard
  - OSHA Tuberculosis Control Guidelines
  - Hazard Communication and Training
  - Material Safety Data Sheets (MSDS)

Place a manual in each work area including the lab, breakroom, etc., so that each employee has quick access to procedural information.

The following examples will give you an idea how these polices should be written. Design the format to suit your practice.

Appointment Scheduling and Registration Policy

Appointments

- The receptionist will make all appointments.
- Scheduling appointments for Dr.________________.
  - New patients are allotted _______ minutes.
  - Routine follow-up appointments are allotted _______ minutes.
  - Regular office revisits are allotted _______ minutes.

- Scheduling appointments for Dr.________________.

    - New patients are allotted _______ minutes.

    - Route follow-up appointments are allotted _______ minutes.

    - Regular office revisits are allotted _______ minutes.

- Do not schedule appointments between _______ and _______ (unless it is an emergency or the only time the patient can be seen), as the doctors have hospital visits to make during these times.

- Appointment schedulers should remind all patients to bring in their current insurance card.

- Each morning the receptionist will make a copy of the appointments scheduled for that day and place it on the doctor's desk.

- The receptionist will add to the doctor's list any added appointments which are made throughout the day.

- When making appointments, list in the book the name of the patient, the phone number, age (if a child), the problem, and whether it is a new patient (N/P). Ask for a daytime phone number as well as home number.

- Other Considerations

    - Allowance in the scheduling system should be made for walk-ins and work-ins.

    - If there is a question concerning the urgency of a patient seeing the doctor before an opening is available, refer the call to the doctor.

    - Call patients the day before to remind them of their appointments. Never leave messages on a recorder or with an individual other than the patient.

- Pulling Patient Charts

    - Patient charts for the next day's scheduled appointments must be pulled each evening and kept in the front office until the patient arrives.

    - A Superbill is placed on the chart. The chart is then placed in a designated location for the medical assistant or nurse.

    - Patient charts are to be returned to the front office for filing.

- Patients will be taken in the order of appointment rather than order of arrival unless their illness warrants immediate attention.

In summary, have a full understanding of office policies as follows:

- Physician's time allotments

    - Telephone calls/professional

    - Meetings

    - Family/friends

    - Social Commitments

- Patient appointment needs

    - Scheduling protocol

    - Ancillary services

- ■ Employee schedules
  - Lunch hours
  - Work area restrictions
- ■ Patient telephone services
  - Prescriptions
  - Counseling concerns/direction
  - Community services

Reception and Registration

- ■ Receptionist greets patients as they arrive. Patients should always be greeted by name.
- ■ All patients should be asked to sign in.
- ■ If it is a new patient, a practice brochure is given to them.
- ■ Patient completes the *Patient Information Registration* form (Exhibit 5-1) if it is a first visit. Assistance should be offered for completing the form. Registration forms should be checked for completeness.
- ■ Superbill — a superbill is prepared (printed) and placed on the patient's chart.
- ■ The receptionist should check the sign-in sheet on a regular basis to assure that no patients have been overlooked.
- ■ If a new patient, ask to see their driver's license and insurance card. Make a copy and put it in the patient's file.
- ■ At each visit, review each managed care enrollee's membership card to assure that coverage is in effect.
- ■ For all patients, reconfirm phone numbers and addresses.

The policies and procedures manual will describe the protocols for each function within the practice. Preparation will require a generous investment in time and effort but will be well worth the effort due to the guidance and training it will provide.

Efficient appointment scheduling is best maintained by using a guide to estimate times.
(See *Guide to Estimated Times for Common Medical Procedures* — Exhibit 5-2. Also, see
Appointment Schedule Form — Exhibit 5-3.)

Facility Management

Office Environment

How do your patients perceive the office environment, and more specifically, the reception area? Is the reception area warm and inviting? Does it have a calming, peaceful atmosphere? Or is it chaotic and noisy? Do patients have "space," or do they feel too close to other "sick" patients? Patients often form judgments about a physician and the practice the moment they walk through the front door. What impression do you give?

Take the time to sit in your reception area for five minutes once a month. Observe everything.
Are the windows and window treatments clean? Is there dust on the tables or woodwork? How
do the plants look? Are the chairs comfortable? Is the upholstery in good condition? You are
seeing what your patients see. Make improvements accordingly.

Some suggestions to create a pleasant reception area include:

- Create a living-room effect.

- Decorate tastefully.

- Use table lamps rather than fluorescent lighting.

- ·Display arrangements of fresh cut flowers.

- Provide educational videos on interesting health topics.

- Provide tasteful distractions such as an aquarium, art objects, wall hangings.

- Play soothing, easy-listening music.

- Give patients something to do, e.g., puzzles, books, current magazines, patient education
  brochures.

Facility Management

If your medical practice is located in a freestanding office building, make sure the building,
parking lot and offices are clean and in good repair. The common grounds should be well-
landscaped and maintained. Create a good impression for the patient.

Consider your overall building and grounds needs and develop a program for facility maintenance.
Weigh the pros and cons of having a year-round service by a landscape company versus hiring a
reliable individual to do general lawn care and maintenance. A student or retired person who is
capable of yard work, janitorial service, and minor repairs may offer a wider range of services at a
lower cost than a service company. Whomever you hire, be sure to have a detailed checklist of the
services you expect and monitor the results on a monthly basis.

Landscape and janitorial contractors who have provided services over an extended period tend to
get lax if you do not check what they do. Do not accept less than you pay for from any
contractor who provides services for a price. Let them know you are checking the results of their
work and if their performance is not up to your standards. There is no room for passiveness in
dealing with contractors. Do not accept mediocre service. Consider withholding part of the
payment until contract requirements are met. When negotiating a new contract, be specific about
what you want and spell it out in the contract.

The Physical Plant

The design and layout of the medical office should be functional for the physician and office
staff, and comfortable and safe for patients.

The reception area is the first link in the marketing effort — the patient's first impression of the
practice. It should be clean and uncluttered. Seating should be comfortable with allowances
made for patients with special needs (such as the elderly or disabled patients). If children are
frequently present in the reception area, provide a "play area." Current and varied reading
material should be available.

The appearance of the business office is a reflection of the organization and efficiency of the practice. Work stations should be free of clutter. If storage space is limited and items are stored in boxes or on open shelves, these should be neat, well-arranged, and out of the sight of the patient.

A clear glass window as the check-in point ensures confidentiality when discussing sensitive matters.

Exam and treatment rooms should be clean and well stocked. Arrange common items the same in all examination rooms. Store hazardous chemicals and/or equipment in a cabinet or storage closet. Include a mirror and extra hooks in exam rooms for patients to hang clothing when they disrobe.

Ensure that signs are clear, large enough to be seen, and well-placed, with nothing obstructing the view.

Evaluate the adequacy of parking facilities for patient flow. Parking lots should be well-located, well-marked, and well-lit. The American with Disabilities Act (ADA) requires that employers and service providers accommodate the disabled with designated parking space. Make sure your facility meets the requirements.

Evaluation of the physical facility every six months ensures that the facility meets the appropriate standards.

Following is a checklist for evaluating the interior office and facility premises.

Interior Office Checklist

	YES	NO
1. Magazines current (none older than 30 days), in good condition (crisp, without rips or tears), appropriate for target market.	❑	❑
2. Patient information material current, in good supply.	❑	❑
3. Patient entertainment material current, in good supply, and appropriate for target market.	❑	❑
4. Chairs, sofas, and tables clean and in excellent repair.	❑	❑
5. Individual chairs with firm arm rests, rather than seating joined at the arms.	❑	❑
6. Seating arranged so that strangers facing one another are at least eight feet apart.	❑	❑
7. Windows clean.	❑	❑
8. Draperies clean, hanging straight.	❑	❑
9. Carpets clean and in good repair (no threadbare spots) without stains, holes, frays along binding, or bubbles.	❑	❑
10. Uncovered floors spotless.	❑	❑
11. Restrooms clean with toilet tissue in good supply.	❑	❑
12. Reception or waiting areas free from medicine odors.	❑	❑
13. Pictures and wall hangings: glass clean, frames hanging straight, appropriate to office image.	❑	❑
14. Walls, wallpaper, and cabinets clean of smudges or marks, without unsightly chips, and moldings dusted.	❑	❑
15. Waiting room large enough to accommodate patient load. Doors easy to open, close completely and securely.	❑	❑
16. Examination rooms soundproof.	❑	❑
17. Temperatures in all areas within acceptable ranges for patients.	❑	❑
18. Office plants alive, dusted, pruned, watered.	❑	❑
19. Examination rooms spotless, tidy, equipment in good repair, modern-looking.	❑	❑
20. Examination table covers: no rips or frays.	❑	❑
21. Doctor's office clean, dusted, tidy, and orderly.	❑	❑
(Other)____	❑	❑
(Other)____	❑	❑

Inspected by:____

Signed:____ Date:___________________

Facility Evaluation

Comments   *YES*   *NO*

1. Do exterior signs serve to attract patients to your practice?   ☐   ☐   ______

2. Do signs communicate a caring, professional image?   ☐   ☐   ______

3. Is the outside approach (hallways, sidewalk, foyer) clean, well-lit, clear of obstacles?   ☐   ☐   ______

4. Is the parking facility adequate?

5. Are handicapped spaces near the building and clearly marked?   ☐   ☐   ______

6. Is your practice location conveniently accessible to the majority of your patients?   ☐   ☐   ______

7. Is your practice convenient to the emergency room and other facilities you use?   ☐   ☐   ______

8. Is your practice convenient to major traffic arteries and public transportation?   ☐   ☐   ______

9. Does traffic congestion hinder accessibility to your parking area?   ☐   ☐   ______

10. Does your location allow for facility expansion?   ☐   ☐   ______

11. Is your facility accessible to ambulances?   ☐   ☐   ______

12. Is landscaping maintained in each season?   ☐   ☐   ______

13. Does the main building entrance have doors that open automatically?   ☐   ☐   ______

14. Is the building directory immediately obvious upon building entry?   ☐   ☐   ______

15. Can the receptionist see the entire reception area?   ☐   ☐   ______

16. Is there sufficient space for writing on the patient side of the check-in and check-out counters?   ☐   ☐   ______

17. Is there a place to hang coats?   ☐   ☐   ______

18. Are restroom facilities adequate?   ☐   ☐   ______

19. Is there a need for a diaper changing area in the restroom?   ☐   ☐   ______

20. Do restrooms accommodate the handicapped?   ☐   ☐   ______

21. Is the reception desk visible upon entry to the office?   ☐   ☐   ______

CHAPTER 6

Managed Care

Practice Enhancement

The rapidly changing health care environment is challenging practitioners to develop more efficient systems of medical practice management and to cultivate patient relationships through adopting marketing strategies, not only to attract new patients, but to maintain the loyalties of existing patients.

With increasing competition, decreasing reimbursement, and rising costs to operate a medical practice, a practitioner cannot afford to be a passive participant in this dynamic environment.

In order to effectively develop practice building strategies, it is important to understand the chief characteristics of the health care consumer. Without this foundation to build on, a practitioner may miss the most obvious opportunities for practice enhancement.

Patient Satisfaction Survey

To measure changes in patient opinions over time, conduct surveys at four-month, six-month, or twelve-month intervals. The questionnaire must be the same for each survey for the answers to be comparable. However, you may ask additional questions at the end of each survey of interest at that time.

By using yes and no answers on your survey, tabulating results is quicker, easier, and more consistent. Prioritize the results/comments. If a majority of the respondents say they are not being seen on time, that issue needs to be addressed first. If a majority of patients say they are considering a physician in another location because of parking fees, respond by implementing validated parking. Notify patients of your response, and thank them for their feedback.

Development

Use a pre-printed survey or develop your own. If you develop your own survey, the following survey questions are suggested:

	YES	NO	
1. Do you feel you understand the specialty of our practice?	❑	❑	_________
2. Do you believe you are aware of all the services we offer?	❑	❑	_________
3. Is the location of our office convenient?	❑	❑	_________
4. Do you find our waiting room comfortable?	❑	❑	_________

	YES	**NO**	

5. Do you feel relaxed in the waiting room? ☐ ☐ _______

6. Are our parking facilities adequate? ☐ ☐ _______

7. Is having to pay for parking a hindrance to receiving your care here? ☐ ☐ _______

8. Do you have to pay to park when you see other practitioners? ☐ ☐ _______

9. What changes would you make in the physical aspects of our office? ☐ ☐ _______

____

____

10. Do you find our front office personnel (secretary, receptionist, etc.)

Friendly? ☐ ☐ _______

Courteous? ☐ ☐ _______

Efficient? ☐ ☐ _______

11. Do you find our business personnel (practice administrator, bookkeeper, etc.)

Friendly? ☐ ☐ _______

Courteous? ☐ ☐ _______

Efficient? ☐ ☐ _______

12. Are your phone calls handled in a prompt, courteous manner? ☐ ☐ _______

13. Are you receiving adequate help with your insurance? ☐ ☐ _______

14. Have you received a copy of our business policies? ☐ ☐ _______

15. Have our payment and billing policies been explained to your satisfaction? ☐ ☐ _______

16. Do you find our nurses

Friendly? ☐ ☐ _______

Courteous? ☐ ☐ _______

Efficient? ☐ ☐ _______

17. Do you feel our nurses are sympathetic to your illness? ☐ ☐ _______

18. Do you find the doctor(s):

Friendly? ☐ ☐ _______

Courteous? ☐ ☐ _______

Efficient? ☐ ☐ _______

YES   NO

19. Do you feel the doctor is interested in you as a person?

20. Does the doctor spend enough time with you?

21. Is your wait too long in the reception area before you see the doctor?

22. Do you have to wait too long in the examination room before you see the doctor?

23. Is our answering service prompt and courteous?

24. Do our doctors promptly return your calls?

25. Are your phone calls to the doctors during the day?

26. Do you mind if the nurses respond to some of your calls?

27. Are you satisfied with the hospital we use?

28. Is this hospital convenient for you and your family?

29. Do you feel that our fees are:

    High?

    Average?

30. Have you used other health services (such as an emergency clinic) because you felt it would be less expensive? If yes, which one(s)?

____

____

31. Do you have trouble getting an appointment as soon as you would like?

32. Are our secretaries helpful in finding appointments that meet your needs?

33. Are our office hours convenient for you? If no, how could we best serve you?

____

____

34. Would you like more educational information from us?

35. If we have audiovisual tapes available about your medical problem, would you use them?

36. Would you want to receive a health newsletter from us
periodically? ☐ ☐ __________

37. How were you referred to this practice? ☐ ☐ __________

☐ Other patients   ☐ Friends   ☐ Yellow Pages
☐ Medical society   ☐ Another doctor   ☐ Our reputation

Other:____

38. Are you satisfied enough with the care we provide to
refer other people to us? ☐ ☐ __________

Comments: ____

____

____

____

____

____

____

____

____

____

____

____

____

(See *Patient Satisfaction Survey Form* — Exhibit 6-1.)

Patient Services and Amenities

Following are some additional value-added services you can provide for your patients:

- Assign someone in your office the responsibility of managing the practice's relationships with its most important customers the patients.

- Send a welcome letter to a patient after the initial appointment has been made. Thank the patient and enclose a practice brochure.

- Acknowledge patients immediately upon arrival.

- Always address a patient by name. Be very sensitive to the patient's feelings about the use of formal or informal terms of address.

- Explain all lengthy delays, and make sure that patients are given the opportunity to reschedule if they so desire. The physician should be encouraged to be punctual and attentive to the appointment schedule. Remember, the patient's time is valuable, too!

- Let disabled or elderly patients know that by prearrangement they can be met at their cars and escorted into the office. Have a wheelchair available.

- Provide child care services. Incorporate babysitting or day care services into your practice, or locate in an area where such services are readily available.

- Provide full-service assistance. Larger multi-specialty groups might employ a "referral coordinator" to help patients choose the appropriate specialist. This individual may also handle appointment scheduling, collection of "pre-visit" information, and answer financial and insurance questions.

- Provide educational materials. Usually "educated" patients are more able and willing to assume responsibility for assisting in the healing process. Many forms of patient education are available; for example, you may write your own educational materials, produce your own video or audio cassettes, establish a lending library, provide preprinted forms, etc.

- Ask about the patient's family. Some physicians jot down personal notes about each patient and keep them in the patient's chart. A few physicians even have photographs taken of each patient and attach them to charts to refresh the physician's memory.

- Spend adequate time with each patient. Surveys indicate that patient satisfaction is directly correlated with the amount of time the physician spends with the patient.

- Answer patients' questions. The basic questions that must be answered are: What is wrong with me? What caused it? What are you and I going to do about it? How long is it going to take? How much is it going to cost? What effect will it have on activities?

- Maintain eye contact with your patients while you are talking to them.

- Never interrupt or contradict a patient's objections. Instead, listen, restate, paraphrase and explain.

- Explain the necessity of all lab tests and X-ray examinations you order and the billing procedures for such examinations.

- Inform patients about what happens after they leave. Let them know what you will be doing for them before their next visit, and that you will follow the progress of their cases.

- Walk patients to the door, or in some other way bring your encounter with the patient to a cordial conclusion.

- When appropriate, call patients a few days after their visit to see how they are doing. Most patients will greatly appreciate your concern.

- Call with good lab results. Patients appreciate knowing all is well.

- Send holiday cards, birthday cards, etc.

- Send flowers to a new mother, or treat the new parents to dinner.

- Stamp "thank you" on the face of all patients' canceled checks.

- Schedule follow-up visits and use a tickler system for reminder cards. Do not tell a patient to call for an appointment in six months and assume the patient will.

- Send reminders for annual health care visits. A reminder system can be set up and might be coordinated with the patient's birthday so that a combination birthday card/reminder notice can be sent.

Marketing in a Managed Care Market

Although managed care is having an effect on marketing, do not give up on those tried and true strategies that worked so well in the fee-for-service environment. Many of them will still be useful in a managed care setting and can help you achieve a successful marketing strategy in the transition period. As long as fee for service represents a substantial percentage of revenue, continue to actively market for that population. The vast majority of providers nationwide derive at least 90 percent of their revenues from fee-for-service encounters. It is important not to neglect the indemnity market.

Marketing decisions are being based on what the market will look like several years in the future in a managed care marketplace. However, during this time of transition, it is not only possible but important to engage in marketing activities that are productive both in the indemnity market and in the managed care market.

In most markets, for probably several years yet, there is more indemnity than there is managed care business. Continue to advertise in the yellow pages advertising and use other forms of promotion to increase your market share. The future will bring a real battle for indemnity business, so prepare now for leaner times.

The question is when is the time to reduce marketing activities for indemnity business and transfer to managed care organizations. Patient satisfaction is critical as managed care becomes more dominate in the market. Practices, therefore, must prepare satisfaction surveys and monitor patient satisfaction.

There is a substantial difference between maintaining patient satisfaction in managed care versus fee-for-service. For example, under managed care, if five percent of your patients express their dissatisfaction to the payer, you could lose 100 percent of the patients from that plan if the contract is not renewed. Therefore, patient satisfaction, while important before, will have significant financial impact in the future. Satisfaction surveys should not only target your patients, but also your referral relationships.

Ten Ways to Show Health Plans How Good You Are

Set up a file labeled *quality.* In it, file in all the credentials, minutes, plans, and memos that you generate. Consider these steps.

- Keep minutes of office staff meetings.
- Improve clinical recordkeeping.
- Conduct patient satisfaction surveys.
- Set up treatment protocols.
- Identify your most common diagnoses.
- See how you compare to other doctors in cost, quality, access.
- Keep track of the time you certify disability for a given diagnosis.
- Make your practice *patient friendly.*
- Tell payers, referring physicians, and patients about your efforts.

Strategies for the Managed Care Marketplace

- Accept the inevitability of managed care.
- Strengthen your network (MDs, hospitals).
- Cultivate third party payer relationships.
- Obtain discounted fee-for-service contracts before capitated contracts.
- Maintain membership in more than one plan.
- Know the contract before you sign it.
- Learn how to negotiate.
- Consider employment of physician extenders.
- Maintain up-to-date contract reference files.
- Develop internal quality control procedures.
- Control practice overhead.
- Become proactive.

The Health Plan Profile

The Health Plan Profile is an example of a helpful and timesaving tool for the receptionist and for the employee responsible for pre-authorization or test scheduling.

The profile provides employees with a "quick reference" to the various requirements of the managed care plans that are accepted by the practice.

Prepare a profile for each plan and place in three-ring binders. Keep one at the front desk and another where it is accessible to the employee scheduling tests or pre-authorizations. The binder allows for easy up-dates and additions. Since it will be used repeatedly, the pages should have reinforced holes or sheet protectors. (See *Health Plan Profile* — Exhibit 6-2.)

Tracking Pre-Certification

It is always wise to have in place a plan for tracking pre-certification information. In the event a pre-certification is challenged, you will have a record of who authorized the procedure. The following method of tracking may be helpful to you:

- Use a colored or fluorescent paper for easy identification.
- Use two forms to a page (make each form 8"x 5").
- Reprint the form with the following headings:
  - Patient name
  - Managed care plan name
  - Appointment date
  - Diagnosis
  - Procedure
  - Provider
  - Name of person who gave the pre-certification authorization.

Telephone Triage Guidelines

Provide the instructions your staff needs by setting up a written telephone protocol. Having a written telephone protocol provides a degree of malpractice protection. Your manual is evidence that employees are not giving advice off the cuff; instead, they are following your approved guidelines. Similarly, telephone protocol finds favor with managed care plans because of their concerns with quality and patient satisfaction.

How to write a telephone protocol manual

- *Standardize the guidelines.* Reach agreement with your partners and your nurses on how to handle conditions and symptoms commonly encountered. Avoid having different protocols that frustrate staff and upset patients. Prepare a draft and have the physicians and the rest of the clinical staff check for loopholes or to uncover the need for clarifications.

- *Make the manual user-friendly.* Arrange each condition or system (ear, head, heart, nose, etc.) alphabetically, followed by your specific scheduling guidelines. Include a short list of questions under each heading to elicit details of the patient's symptoms.

  Include all the conditions you deal with frequently. Attach an alphabetical index and number the pages. Preface the manual with a few pages on telephone courtesy and your general policies for giving advice and authorizing prescription renewals.

  When needed, update the manual with additions and revisions. Keep the pages in a three-ring binder so you can replace them easily. Put a copy of the manual near each phone in the office. Remember to date each revision.

- *Post your emergency instructions prominently.* On a separate sheet, list medical emergencies such as chest pain, heavy bleeding, fainting, seizure, and poisoning (include the phone number of the local poison control center) and post a copy near each telephone. Route these calls to a physician immediately.

  If no doctor is available, the patient should be directed to the nearest emergency room. Call an ambulance if he cannot get there on his own and arrange for a doctor to meet him at the hospital. Do not put anyone on hold if an emergency is suspected. Ask for the caller's phone number in case you are disconnected. (Do not put callers on hold without asking first if they will hold. Simply answering, "Doctor's office — hold please" is not acceptable.)

  Test your system by checking how well your employees handle emergencies. Doctors and nurses can pose as callers and put the staff through some hypothetical situations to ensure that the protocols are adequate and that everyone is confident in following them.

- *Limit your malpractice risk.* If a patient wants medical advice, the call should be put through to a nurse or other medical professional; only the most critical calls should be routed to the doctors. When in doubt, nurses or PAs should not hesitate to get a physician.

  It is a clear malpractice risk to let unlicensed employees give clinical advice, however simple and straightforward it may seem. Never should a non-clinical employee give medical advice or attempt to answer a patient's questions about symptoms.

  State in your personnel manual that any attempt by unauthorized personnel to give advice or answer clinical questions will be grounds for immediate termination. Your reputation, patients' safety, and your exposure to malpractice liability ride on the accuracy of information that patients receive.

There is risk of being dropped from an insurer's panel if your managed care plan discovers that an unlicensed employee is giving medical advice.

- **Do not expect to always go "by the book."** Though you want to avoid unnecessary visits, be flexible. While many patients just call for reassurance, some will insist on coming to the office. Whoever takes the call should schedule the appointment and note the conversation in the patient's chart so the doctor will be aware of previous contact. Similarly, if a patient thinks he should be scheduled sooner rather than later, even for something as simple as a cold, put the call through to a triage nurse. If a nurse is not available to take the call, the person answering should take a message and route it to a nurse or physician, along with the chart.

- **Pay attention to routine calls.** Return all calls promptly. Tell patients to call the office any time if their symptoms worsen. Assure your patients that they will not be a bother and instruct them to call if they have any doubts. Give patients the name of your triage nurse, and encourage them to contact this staff member first.

Document all calls that need to be returned. Include the patient's name, phone numbers, the time and date, the nature of the complaint, any medications being taken, and the initials of whoever took the call. Record any advice given, and put the completed message sheet in the patient's chart.

Block out an hour each day for calls that must be personally returned or handle callbacks a few at a time between patients. Get back to patients on the same day.

If you use an answering machine for after hours calls, make sure your message gives a number where you can be reached in a crisis. Your message should also say that a doctor or nurse will return non-urgent calls as soon as possible. Patients are not pleased if your message just states your office hours and simply says to dial 911 or head for the ER in an emergency.

CHAPTER 7

Risk Management in the Medical Office

There has been a steady increase in the number of medical malpractice claims over the past ten years. The causes of these lawsuits can generally be attributed to the following:

- Scientific advances that enable cures for certain previously untreatable conditions but, at the same time, carry inherent risks of undesirable results or side effects.

- "The Marcus Welby Syndrome" — unrealistic expectations of what can be done. Many people still expect a *cure* for every ailment.

- Reduced communication between physician and patient and the subsequent breakdown of personal rapport.

- An increasingly lawsuit-oriented society that seeks to hold someone at fault for injuries or accidents that previously were considered misfortune.

Developing a Loss Prevention Program

Any effective program of loss prevention must emphasize risk management and quality assurance. The physician and administrator must set into action a plan to:

- Identify existing or potential patient care problems.

- Establish criteria for patient care responsibility.

- Measure and monitor the actual performance of the staff.

- Investigate and resolve problems or complaints.

- Monitor the corrective action.

- Educate employees about government regulatory programs and the recordkeeping requirements for each program.

- Provide continuing education for both employees and patients.

The remainder of this chapter addresses each area of practice operation individually and provides suggestions for developing loss prevention protocol in these areas.

Scheduling

A common source of patient dissatisfaction in a physician's office is the length of time the patient must wait once arriving at the office. When they endure long waits, patients perceive a lack of concern. When there is a dissatisfied patient, the risk of a professional liability claim increases. Consider these points when scheduling patients.

- The length of time it takes to get an appointment.

- The receptionist's demeanor.

- When calling for an appointment, if patients are asked permission before being put on hold.
- The average length of time a patient is left on hold on the telephone.

The maximum time a patient should wait in the reception area is thirty minutes. If the wait is any longer, he or she becomes dissatisfied. To decrease the patient's wait time, we recommend the following:

- Schedule extra time for new patients or special procedures.
- Provide enough time before and after seeing patients. Avoid over-booking patients.
- Inform patients of any delays in the appointment schedule and the cause for the delay.
- Call patients at home to advise them of any expected delays.
- Block off time each day for walk-ins and emergencies. Fill these times no earlier than the evening before.

Documentation of appointment information is almost as critical as the progress note itself. Always document. The following guidelines should be used in appointment documentation.

- Record missed or cancelled appointments in the patient's chart.
- Do not erase, white out or otherwise obliterate any appointment in the appointment book or computer schedule.
- Document any attempts to reach the patient to reschedule a missed appointment. If the patient's condition warrants, send a certified letter.

Billing and Collections

Many malpractice claims are initiated in response to the manner in which collection efforts are made. A written collections policy assures that all employees know what the policy is and how to handle each billing and collection situation. Consider addressing these issues in your policy:

- Letting the patient know before his first appointment about your fee and payment requirements.
- A review procedure for circumstances that require special action.
- The patient's past payment history.
- The quality of care.
- The patient's satisfaction. If the patient balks at paying a bill, discuss it. Work out an agreeable payment arrangement, if possible.
- The cost of legal action versus the amount of money owed. Obtain information from the appropriate small claims court in your area.
- Having the physician review every chart before initiating aggressive collection procedures.
- Understanding of patient's rights concerning privacy and the physician-patient relationship. (Do not send any medical information to a collection agency.)
- Awareness of Fair Debt Collection Act. (Periodically evaluate the collection agency's practices.)

Environment

The patient develops a first impression of the kind of medical care he will receive when he views the practice surroundings. If the environment is pleasant, clean and convenient, the physician will be more likely to be viewed as competent and providing quality care.

- To prevent patient injury, evaluate the facility to ensure easy access. All patient care areas should be checked, including the parking lot, to identify any potential safety hazards.

- Provide comfortable office furnishing to allow the patient to feel at ease. Check furnishings periodically to assure that they are in good condition. Take steps to ensure cleanliness and good housekeeping. Messy or dirty offices create a negative impression. The effect on perceived quality is significant.

- Have furnishings that meet the needs of various patients. Soft and/or low seating is problematic for pregnant women, the elderly and the infirm.

- Keep the room at a comfortable temperature and provide plenty of lighting.

Medical Equipment

Patients are often injured because of faulty or improper use of equipment. The practice administrator should institute a policy of regular maintenance and use of all equipment.

- Train all employees on the proper use of equipment.

- Document the training and place in each employee's personnel file.

- Calibrate all equipment as recommended by the manufacturer.

- Maintain a log of all equipment maintenance and service.

- Report any patient injury associated with a piece of equipment to your malpractice insurance carrier. Remove the equipment and all its collateral equipment from service.

- Avoid tampering with the equipment or sending it to the manufacturer for repair until the insurance company has been notified and you are instructed to do so.

- ***Do not document any assumptions about equipment malfunction or improper usage in the medical record.***

Emergencies

All medical offices should have a written protocol for handling a patient emergency.

- Post all emergency numbers such as ambulance, hospital, poison control etc., next to all telephones.

- Require all staff to stay current on cardiopulmonary resuscitation (CPR).

- If the office has emergency equipment and/or medications, all staff should be trained to use such equipment and drugs. It is better not to have this equipment on hand than to have untrained employees using it. There is often less liability in doing nothing than in doing something incorrectly.

- Conduct periodic emergency drills.

Confidentiality

Communication between the patient and physician is confidential. Patient confidentiality is critical to the patient/doctor relationship. Many suits have been filed due to breach of confidential information. It is the patient's right to decide what information may be revealed to others. This confidentiality privilege extends to all members of the health care team.

- All personal data, medical notes *and* billing information is confidential and may not be communicated to anyone without the patient's written consent.

- Do not discuss a patient's illness with any staff member who does not need to know.

- Do not discuss a patient's illness with family members or friends except in the presence of and with the consent of the patient.

- Loose talk that is overheard by others can be the basis for a defamation or invasion of privacy suit. Watch your voice volume; pay attention to who is nearby.

- Do a "confidentiality audit" of your office. Test to see how easy it is to overhear conversations. If you need to, install some sound proofing.

- Avoid discussing a patient's medical care on a cellular phone with either the patient or anyone else. These conversations are sometimes picked up by police scanners and radios.

- Discuss confidentiality issues with all new employees. Make sure all staff members understand that violation of a patient's privacy is grounds for termination. Staff members should, at the time of hiring, sign a form pledging confidentiality of patient information, and this form should be a part of the personnel record.

Handling Patient Complaints

A patient indicates dissatisfaction and intentions to sue long before the legal papers are served. A staff member may be the first to be aware of a patient complaint. Regardless of how minor they may seem, *all complaints* need to be brought to the physician's attention.

- Institute a formal complaint policy in the office. Use an incident report form and a complaint log to track the occurrence and disposition of all patient complaints. (See *Incident Report Form* — Exhibit 7-1. Also, see *Patient Complaint Log* — Exhibit 7-2.)

- Notify the physician of the complaint on the day it is received.

- Respond to the complaint quickly and follow up with the patient. To assure that they are satisfied with the solution, document the contact in the medical record.

Termination of the Patient/Physician Relationship.

The implied contract between a patient and a physician begins *not* when an appointment is made, but when examination or treatment begins.

Once a physician-patient relationship has been established, the physician is not free to terminate the relationship at will without formal, written notification. The physician-patient relationship continues until it is ended by one of the following circumstances:

- The patient has no need of further care.

- The patient terminates the relationship.

- The physician formally terminates the relationship.

Failure to terminate may constitute patient abandonment and bring about fines or legal action if the patient is harmed by the abandonment.

There may be several occasions when it will become necessary to terminate the physician-patient relationship. Perhaps the patient is noncompliant, and it is believed that continued treatment would increase the chances of a complication or poor outcome. Perhaps the patient is rude or abusive, or maybe the physician and the patient just do not get along. Any of those reasons, and many others, may be a reason to terminate a patient from your practice. If you do so, be sure to follow some specific guidelines to minimize the chance of being sued for abandonment.

A physician *cannot* refuse to give a patient an appointment because the patient has not paid the bill without first terminating the physician-patient relationship. This can be accomplished by sending the patient a *certified, return receipt letter.*

- First, put the notice in writing. The reason may or may not be stated.
  - If for noncompliance, say so clearly in the letter.
  - If for personality conflict, an unpaid bill, or for a reason not to be made public, avoid stating the reason in writing.
- Send the letter by certified mail, return receipt requested. Keep the receipt in the patient's file, along with a copy of the letter.

The amount of time that you are required to give a patient to seek alternative healthcare varies in each state. You are advised to contact your local medical society or attorney to find an answer. This termination process protects you from having to see the patient who fails to follow your suggested treatment plan.

The physician-patient relationship is the foundation of medical law. Upon it rests the legal rights and obligations of both patients and physicians.

(See *Sample Discharge Letter* — Exhibit 7-3.)

Rights of the Patient:

- The right to choose the physician from whom he or she wishes to receive treatment.
- The right to say whether or not medical treatment will begin and to set limits on the care provided.
- The right to know before the treatment begins what it will consist of, what effect it will have on the body, what the inherent dangers are, and what it will cost.

Consent to Treatment

Legal consequences for treating a patient without properly informed consent include charges of assault and battery and negligence.

- Treating a patient without permission is grounds for an assault and battery charge.
- Treating a patient with the patient's consent but failing to explain the inherent risks of a procedure could result in a charge of negligence.

Implied consent is reflected in the patient's actions such as having a prescription filled or accepting an injection.

Expressed consent is an oral or written acceptance of the treatment. The written form of expressed consent is recommended when the proposed treatment involves surgery, experimental drugs or procedures, or high-risk diagnostic or treatment procedures.

Informed Consent to Treatment

The fiduciary relationship between physician and patient is based on trust and confidence. The nature of this relationship obligates the physician to act for the benefit of the patient.

Contained in this obligation is the physician's duty to voluntarily inform the patient of all relevant information concerning the treatment being offered including potential hazards and risks. This duty and legal principle that a mentally competent adult has control over his/her own body requires a physician to obtain the patient's informed consent before beginning medical treatment.

Informed consent will develop from the patient's understanding of the:

- General nature of the treatment and consequences involved.
- Normal risks and hazards of inherent treatment.
- Side effects or complications that are known to occur.
- Alternative treatments.

Patient's Obligations

- The obligation to tell the physician the truth about the nature and duration of his or her symptoms and to provide medical history.
- The obligation to follow the physician's instructions concerning diet, medication, exercise, habits, follow-up appointments, etc.
- The obligation to pay the physician for services rendered.

Physician's Obligations

- The obligation to treat the patient as long as the patient's condition requires it, or until a proper withdrawal or discharge is made.
- The obligation to inform patients of proposed treatment and to obtain appropriate consent before proceeding.
- The obligation to caution patients against unneeded or undesirable surgery.
- The obligation to provide complete and accurate instructions to the patient and, when applicable, to the person responsible for the patient in the physician's absence.
- The obligation to respect the patient's privacy and confidential information acquired during the course of the physician-patient relationship.

A Physician is NOT obligated to:

- Accept new patients or former patients with new problems.
- Demonstrate perfect or infallible judgment, acquire a maximum level of skill, or obtain the maximum amount of education.
- Diagnose correctly every medical problem or cure each patient. Lack of skill on the physician's part cannot be assumed simply because a patient does not recover.
- Return a patient to the state of health experienced before the patient became ill or injured.
- Know in advance how each patient will respond to every drug or anesthesia.
- Continue treating a patient who has discharged the physician, even if the patient later experiences adverse effects.

The Medical Record

A well documented, legible, structured medical record is the physician's first line of defense in the event of a malpractice suit. The medical record is a form of communication among health care professionals about the patient's condition. This documentation identifies the patient, supports the diagnosis, justifies the treatment and documents the results of treatment.

The medical record is confidential. The information is private, should remain secure and should not be made public. The record belongs to the physician, but the information belongs to the patient.

Authorization to Release Records

The patient has the *sole* authority to release information from his medical record.

The office should be prepared with a printed release form that the patient signs to release the medical record to a third party. (See *Authorization for Release of Medical Records*, Exhibit 7-4.) The release form need not be complicated or full of legal language.

A word of caution. HIV/AIDS information is *not* included in a standard release form. The release form must *specifically* state that this information is included.

Any mention of HIV/AIDS testing or treatment is extremely sensitive and should be maintained in a separate part of the medical record. Some attorneys suggest it should be maintained in an envelope marked, *CONFIDENTIAL! DO NOT RELEASE.*

TIP: Never release a patient record without the physician's approval.

Records are the heart of systematic patient care. Excellent recordkeeping is one of the most effective tools in patient care and in preventing claims. Following are the key elements of a good medical record. (See *Medical Records Checklist*, Exhibit 7-5.)

- *Uniform Records.* Medical records should be uniform within the practice. Inserting dividers for lab, x-ray, progress notes, etc., and using a problem list is an excellent way to structure charts in a format that organizes the record for easy scanning by all health care professionals who subsequently use the chart. (See *Medical Record Form*, Exhibit 7-6.)

- *Secure Pages.* Secure all pages of the record in chronological order with fasteners to prevent pages from being lost.

- *Organization.* Organize records for easy and accurate retrieval. Whatever system is used, it should be logical and clear to all staff members and physicians (active versus inactive patients; color coding for chronic problems or frequent diagnoses, etc.).

- *Timeliness.* Make all entries in the record, whether written or dictated, at the time of the patient contact. Include the date and the time of the exam or contact. The greater the time lapse between the exam and the entry, the less credible the medical record becomes.

- *Legible Records.* Records must be legible. Health care professionals with illegible handwriting should dictate their notes. This helps to avoid misinterpretations that result in improper treatment.

- **Dictated Records.** Dictated notes must be proofread and signed. The statement "dictated but not read" does not relieve the physician from responsibility for what was transcribed. At best, the statement alerts another health care professional that the note has not been proofed and may not be correct.

- **Accurate Records.** It is important to record all information in objective and concise terms. Never include extraneous information or subjective assessments of the patient, such as "this patient is a jerk." Include direct quotations from the patient. However, reduce the essential information to the least possible number of words.

- **Corrections.** *Never* improperly or unlawfully alter a medical record. If an error has been made, draw a single line through the inaccurate entry and enter the necessary correction. Date, time and initial the correction in the margin. It is also acceptable to make an addendum to a medical record. It should be made after the last entry noting the current date and time, and both entries should be cross-referenced. A record that appears to have been altered implies that a cover-up has occurred. Do not obliterate an entry with a marker or white-out.

- **Jousting.** *Never* criticize or make derogatory comments about another health care professional or organization to the patient or in the medical record. A negative comment can undermine a patient's confidence in the previous health care worker and contribute to or cause a decision to pursue a legal claim regardless of causation and/or who was responsible.

- **Patient Telephone Calls.** Document all patient telephone calls in the medical record. When the physician speaks to a patient while away from the office and the medical record is not available, notes regarding any prescriptions or medical advice given over the telephone can be recorded on a phone call pad. The sheet can be torn out and presented for entry into the chart when the physician returns to the office.

- **Conversations.** Address and document all patient/family worries or concerns in the patient record. Record the source of the information, if other than the patient.

  Always document important warnings and instructions given to the patient at the time of discharge. Documenting discharge instructions may help prove noncompliance. Juries are not as sympathetic of noncompliant patients.

  To reinforce the signed informed consent form, always document information disclosed during the informed consent process.

- **Potential Complications.** Document all possible complications that might occur. Failure to recognize a complication in time to prevent injury is a common basis for lawsuit. Proving negligence is difficult if the record shows prior awareness that a complication might occur.

Exhibits

■ *Monthly Statistics Form* *1*

■ *Employee Safety Orientation Checklist* *2-1*

■ *Accident/Injury Report Employer* *2-2*

■ *Accident/Injury Report Employee* *2-3*

■ *Accident/Injury Report Witness* *2-4*

■ *Exposure Incident Protocol* *2-5*

■ *Exposure Incident Report* *2-6*

■ *Post Exposure Incident Form (Source)* *2-7*

■ *Post Exposure Incident Form (Exposed)* *2-8*

■ *Sample Job Descriptions* *3-1, 3-2, 3-3*

■ *Employee Performance Appraisal Form* *3-4*

■ *Salary Change Recommendation* *3-5*

■ *Corrective Action Form* *3-6*

■ *Terminating Employee Checklist* *3-7*

■ *Practice Management Statistics* *4-1*

■ *Major Expenses by Specialty* *4-2*

■ *Petty Cash Fund* *4-3*

■ *Summary Report for Tracking Practice Growth and Profitability* *4-4*

■ *Patient Information Registration Form* *5-1*

■ *Guide to Estimated Times for Common Medical Office Procedures* *5-2*

■ *Appointment Schedule* *5-3*

■ *Patient Satisfaction Survey* *6-1*

■ *Health Plan Profile* *6-2*

■ *Incident Report Form* *7-1*

■ *Patient Complaint Log* *7-2*

■ *Sample Discharge Letter* *7-3*

■ *Authorization for Release of Medical Records* *7-4*

■ *Medical Records Checklist Form* *7-5*

■ *Medication Record Form* *7-6*

MONTHLY STATISTICS FORM

Month:_______________________________

Total Charges: ...._______________________________

Adjustments: ...._______________________________

Net Charges: ...._______________________________

Total Receipts:......................................._______________________________

Adjustments: ...._______________________________

Net Receipts:......................................._______________________________

Total Patients Seen: ...._______________________________

Daily Average: ...._______________________________

Collection Ratio: ...._______________________________

Accounts Receivable: ...._______________________________

Average Per Patient Charge:......................................._______________________________

Average Per Patient Cost: ...._______________________________

Total Monthly Expense:......................................._______________________________

Net Income:......................................._______________________________

EMPLOYEE SAFETY ORIENTATION CHECKLIST

INJURY AND ILLNESS PREVENTION

Employee Name: ____

Title: ____

Is this a new employee?   ❑ Yes   ❑ No

Is this a new job assignment?   ❑ Yes   ❑ No

1. Has the employee received instruction with respect to general safety and health work practices?   ❑ Yes   ❑ No   If yes, when? _______________________

2. Has the employee received instruction on:

   Emergency Procedures?   ❑ Yes   ❑ No

   Injury & Illness Prevention?   ❑ Yes   ❑ No

   Safety Discipline Policy   ❑ Yes   ❑ No

   Hazard Communication?   ❑ Yes   ❑ No

   Hazardous Material Identification System?   ❑ Yes   ❑ No

3. Has the employee received safety training on the hazards specific to his or her job assignment?   ❑ Yes   ❑ No

4. Does the employee have any known illnesses or ailments that will hamper him or her in the performance of the job assignment?   ❑ Yes   ❑ No

5. Does the employee understand that he or she is required to work safely at all times and is responsible for safety while in the facility?   ❑ Yes   ❑ No

6. Has the employee received a copy of the Safe Work Practices and Safety Rules?   ❑ Yes   ❑ No

_______________________________________   _______________

Employee's Signature   Date

_______________________________________   _______________

Instructor's Name   Date

ACCIDENT/INJURY REPORT — EMPLOYER

Date of Accident/Injury: ___/___/___ **Name of Injured Employee:** ___________________________

Job Title: _________________________________ **How long in this position?** _________

Were Paramedics called? ❑ Yes ❑ No

Was employee: ❑ sent to hospital ❑ clinic   Did employee receive first aid? ❑ Yes ❑ No

What was the employee doing when the injury/accident occurred? ___________________________

____

____

Was the employee trained to do this work? ❑ Yes ❑ No

Has the employee performed this work before? ❑ Yes ❑ No   If yes, how often? _____________

How recently was employee assigned to task that gave rise to the accident? _________________

Based on your investigation, how did the accident/injury occur? ___________________________

____

____

Have any similar accidents occurred in the last 12 months? ❑ Yes ❑ No   If yes, how many? _____

What can be done to prevent a similar incident from occurring in the future? _________________

____

____

Have any corrective measures been implemented? ❑ Yes ❑ No

Specify: ____

____

____

Possible Causes of Injury or Illness (check all that apply)

Employer Responsibilities	Employee Responsibilities	Unsafe Equipment or Material	Unsafe Conditions
❑ No instruction given	❑ Haste or short cuts	❑ Inadequate guarding	❑ Poor light
❑ Incomplete instruction	❑ Did not use proper equipment	❑ Defective equipment	❑ Poor ventilation
❑ Lack of enforcement of safe work practices	❑ Did not use safe work practices	❑ Poor design	❑ Congestion
❑ Lack of proper tools or equipment	❑ Horseplay	❑ Other	❑ Improper piling or storing
❑ Equipment in poor condition	❑ Disregarded instruction		❑ Inadequate exits
❑ Lack of safe work practices	❑ Did not pay attention		❑ Obstructed walkways
❑ Haste	❑ Physical condition of employee		❑ Poor housekeeping
❑ Other	❑ Action of another employee		❑ Other
	❑ Other		

This report was prepared by ____

Print Name/Title

____

Signature   Date

ACCIDENT/INJURY REPORT — EMPLOYEE

Note: The purpose of this report is not to assign blame. Rather, we are attempting to find out how the accident/injury occurred so that we can keep it from happening in the future.

Date of
Accident/Injury: ____/____/____ **Name of Injured Employee:** _______________________________

Job Title: ____ **How long in this position?** _________

What were you doing when the injury/accident occurred? ___________________________________

____

Have you performed this work before? ❏ Yes ❏ No   If yes, how often? ___________________

Describe in detail how the accident/injury occurred. _______________________________________

____

What can be done to prevent a similar incident from occurring in the future? ___________________

____

____

Have any corrective measures been implemented? ❏ Yes ❏ No

Specify: ____

____

____

Possible Causes of Injury or Illness (check all that apply)

❏ No instruction given	❏ Haste or short cuts	❏ Inadequate guarding	❏ Poor light
❏ Incomplete instruction	❏ Did not use proper equipment	❏ Defective equipment	❏ Poor ventilation
❏ Lack of enforcement of safe work practices	❏ Did not use safe work practices	❏ Poor design	❏ Congestion
❏ Lack of proper tools or equipment	❏ Horseplay	❏ Other	❏ Improper piling or storing
❏ Equipment in poor condition	❏ Disregarded instruction		❏ Inadequate exits
❏ Lack of safe work practices	❏ Did not pay attention		❏ Obstructed walkways
❏ Haste	❏ Physical condition of employee		❏ Poor housekeeping
❏ Other	❏ Action of another employee		❏ Other
	❏ Other		

____
Signature   Date

ACCIDENT/INJURY REPORT — WITNESS

Note: The purpose of this report is not to assign blame. Rather, we are attempting to find out how the accident/injury occurred so that we can keep it from happening in the future.

Date of Accident/Injury: ____ / ____ / ____ **Name of Injured Employee:** _________________________

Injured Employee Job Title: ____

Your Name: ____

Your Job Title: _______________________________ **How long in this position?** _________

What was the employee doing when the injury/accident occurred?

Have you performed this work before? ❑ Yes ❑ No If yes, how often? _________________

Describe in detail how the accident/injury occurred? _________________________________

____

What can be done to prevent a similar incident from occurring in the future? _______________

____

____

Have any corrective measures been implemented? ❑ Yes ❑ No

Specify: ____

____

____

Possible Causes of Injury or Illness (check all that apply)

❑ No instruction given	❑ Haste or short cuts	❑ Inadequate guarding	❑ Poor light
❑ Incomplete instruction	❑ Did not use proper equipment	❑ Defective equipment	❑ Poor ventilation
❑ Lack of enforcement of safe work practices	❑ Did not use safe work practices	❑ Poor design	❑ Congestion
		❑ Other	❑ Improper piling or storing
❑ Lack of proper tools or equipment	❑ Horseplay		❑ Inadequate exits
❑ Equipment in poor condition	❑ Disregarded instruction		❑ Obstructed walkways
❑ Lack of safe work practices	❑ Did not pay attention		❑ Poor housekeeping
❑ Haste	❑ Physical condition of employee		❑ Other
❑ Other	❑ Action of another employee		
	❑ Other		

____
Signature   Date

EXPOSURE INCIDENT PROTOCOL

1. Upon exposure to blood or other potentially infectious material, the employee will wash hands and any other skin surface that may have been exposed, and will flush with water mucous membranes which may have been in contact with blood or other potentially infectious materials, as soon as feasible after exposure.

2. Following washing/flushing as described above, the employee will report the following incident to Dr. _________________________________ or to _________________________________

   ____

3. Dr. _________________________________ or _________________________________ will make arrangements for post-exposure evaluation and follow-up with (provider) _________________

   ____.

4. Dr._________________________________ or_________________________________ will ensure that the provider is given the information listed on the Post-Exposure Incident Report to Healthcare Provider and a copy of the OSHA regulations.

5. A copy of the written opinion of the health care provider is obtained within 15 days of the medical evaluation.

6. One copy of the written opinion is given to the employee, and a second copy is filed with the employee medical record.

7. The exposure incident is evaluated and a report of the incident is written by_________________

   ____.

EXPOSURE INCIDENT REPORT

Confidential Employee Medical Record

____

Employee Name (Please print)   Date of Incident

____

Social Security Number   Time of Incident

The Incident

What task or procedure was the employee performing at the time of the incident? _______________

____

How did the incident occur? ____

____

____

What type of body fluid was involved in the incident?______________________________________

The route of exposure was:

- Needlestick with contaminated needle to (site)_______________________________________

- Piercing of skin with contaminated sharp to (site) ___________________________________

- Splashing/spraying of potentially infectious material to (site) ___________________________

- Other (describe) ____

____

The following remedial action may reduce the likelihood of similar incidents in the future:_____________

____

____

This recommendation was instituted on _________________(date)

The Source Individual

The identity of the source individual is:　❏ known　　❏ unknown

❏ known to be infected with:　❏ HBV　　❏ HIV

In accordance with applicable State and local laws, is consent required for testing of the source individual's blood?　❏ Yes　　❏ No

If yes, has consent been obtained?　❏ Yes　　❏ No

- If no, attempts to obtain consent must be documented)
- If yes, has specimen been obtained and tested?　❏ Yes　　❏ No
- If yes, results of this test are ____

Employee Status

Was the Employee previously vaccinated against HBV infection?　❏ Yes　　❏ No

Dates: _______________　_______________　_______________

Post-Exposure Evaluation and Follow-up

The employee was referred for post-exposure evaluation and follow-up:

Name of Health Care Professional: ____

Date/Time of Evaluation:____

Have pertinent employee medical records been given to the provider?　❏ Yes　Date? _____________

____　　　Date

Employee signature

____　　　Date

Plan Administrator

POST-EXPOSURE INCIDENT — SOURCE

SOURCE INDIVIDUAL CONSENT FORM

____

Patient Name (please print):   Social Security Number:

Informed Consent to Blood Testing

I have been informed that an individual has been exposed to my blood or body fluids. As a result of the exposure, I have been asked to permit my blood to be tested for HIV (known to cause AIDS) and HBV.

(Check one.)

❏ I hereby give my consent to such testing.

❏ I consent to have my blood tested for HBV, but I decline to have my blood tested for HIV at this time. I understand that by choosing this option, a sample of my blood will be kept for 90 days, during which period I may change my mind and have my blood tested for HIV at that time.

My consent is based on the understanding that:

1. My test results will remain confidential and provided only to those who have a need to know in accordance with current federal, state, and local statutes.

2. I have been provided with information concerning HIV and HBV, and understand the contents thereof.

3. I have been given the opportunity to ask questions concerning HIV and HBV testing.

4. I will receive a copy of all test results.

____

Signed   Date

Employer's Representative

I certify that the above-named individual received a copy of the HIV/HBV information sheets and has had the contents thereof fully explained.

____

Date   Employer s Representative (Please print)

____

Title

____

Signature

This document will be retained in the exposed employee's medical file.

POST-EXPOSURE INCIDENT — EMPLOYEE

EXPOSED EMPLOYEE CONSENT FORM

____   _______________________________
Employee Name (please print)   Social Security Number

Employee Consent to Blood Testing

As a result of my exposure to blood or other potentially infectious material, it is recommended that I have my blood tested for HIV (known to cause AIDS) and HBV.

(Check one.)

❏ I hereby give my consent to such testing.

❏ I consent to have my blood tested for HBV, but I decline to have my blood tested for HIV at this time. I understand that by choosing this option, a sample of my blood will be kept for 90 days, during which period I may change my mind and have my blood tested for HIV at that time.

My consent is based on the understanding that:

1. My test results will remain confidential and provided only to those who have a need to know in accordance with current federal, state, and local statutes.

2. I will be provided with counseling whether the tests are negative or positive.

3. I will be provided with information concerning HIV and HBV, and understand the contents thereof.

4. I will be given the opportunity to ask questions concerning HIV and HBV testing.

5. I have received risk behavior guidelines concerning HIV.

6. I will receive a copy of all test results.

____   _______________________________
Signed   Date

Employer's Representative

I certify that the above-named individual received a copy of the HIV/HBV information sheets and has had the contents thereof fully explained.

____   _______________________________
Date   Employer's Representative (Please print)

____
Title

____
Signature

This document will be retained in the exposed employee's medical file.

Reports To: Practice Administrator

Experience: Two to five years medical office experience desired.
Some computer experience helpful.

Primary Responsibilities:

- Answer telephone, take all incoming messages and appropriately distribute them throughout the practice staff.

- Handle all appointment scheduling.

- Document all patient financial transactions.

- Balance daily journal including proof of posting and accounts receivable balance.

- Complete patient billing cycle as directed.

- Purge medical records as directed by the practice administrator.

Secondary Responsibilities:

- Back up practice administrator during absences or vacations.

- Other job-related tasks as assigned by the practice administrator and physician.

Signed: ____ **Date:** _______________

NOTE: It is advisable to attach a detailed description of daily tasks to be accomplished and how they are to be accomplished.

Reports To: Practice Administrator/Physician

Primary Responsibilities:

Telephone

a.   Check in/out with answering service.

b.   Answer telephones, take incoming messages and distribute appropriately.
Pull chart for each message.

c.   Answer clinical telephone calls/messages and pharmacy phone calls.

Appointment Scheduling

a.   Schedule appointments; keep record of meetings, conferences, and depositions.

b.   Pull and prepare charts for daily appointments. Attach superbill to each chart.

c.   Print daily appointment schedule.

Secondary Responsibilities:

____

____

____

____

____

____

Signed: ____ **Date:** _________________

Reports To: Practice Administrator/Physician

Primary Responsibilities:

- Check supplies for dictation equipment and restock as needed.

- Pull and file charts as necessary.

- Transcribe all dictation, proofread and print letters and envelopes within 48 hours of dictation.

- File all correspondence, reports, etc., in patient charts in designated order after physician has reviewed and initialed.

- Keep a schedule of professional association meetings, speaking engagements, etc., and remind physician of these commitments.

- Assist physician in gathering data for speaking engagements.

- Release records requested by patients, insurance companies, attorneys, etc.

Secondary Responsibilities:

____

____

____

____

____

____

Signed: ____ **Date:** _______________

EMPLOYEE PERFORMANCE APPRAISAL

STRICTLY CONFIDENTIAL	Date of This Report:

Employee Name:	Performance Time Period: From: To:

Department:	Position Title:

Time in This Classification:	Employment Date:

INSTRUCTIONS:

1. All employees should be appraised at least annually.

2. Use in conjunction with the salary review. Salary changes require approval of the manager and physician.

3. Review employee's work performance for the entire period; refrain from basing judgment on recent events or isolated incidents only.

4. Do not allow personal feelings to govern your rating. Disregard your general impression of the employee.

5. Consider the employee on the basis of the standards you expect to be met for the job. Place a check by the area you feel best describes the employee's performance since the last appraisal.

6. Reason must be given for each factor to substantiate area checked.

QUALITY OF WORK — Consider standard of workmanship, accuracy, neatness, skill, thoroughness, economy of materials, organization of job.

❑ Needs much improvement   ❑ Needs improvement   ❑ Satisfactory
❑ Very good   ❑ Outstanding

Reason:____
____
____

VOLUME OF WORK — Consider use of time, the volume of work accomplished and ability to meet schedules under normal conditions.

❑ Needs much improvement   ❑ Needs improvement   ❑ Satisfactory
❑ Very good   ❑ Outstanding

Reason:____
____
____

ADAPTABILITY — Consider ability to meet changing conditions and situations, ease with which the employee learns new duties and assignments.

❑ Needs much improvement   ❑ Needs improvement   ❑ Satisfactory
❑ Very good   ❑ Outstanding

Reason:____
____
____

JUDGMENT — Consider ability to evaluate relative merit of ideas or facts and arrive at sound conclusions, ability to decide correct course of action when some choice can be made.

❑ Needs much improvement   ❑ Needs improvement   ❑ Satisfactory
❑ Very good   ❑ Outstanding

Reason:____
____
____

JOB KNOWLEDGE AND SKILL — Consider understanding of job procedures and methods, ability to acquire necessary skills, expertise in doing assigned tasks and utilization of background for job.

❑ Needs much improvement   ❑ Needs improvement   ❑ Satisfactory
❑ Very good   ❑ Outstanding

Reason:____
____
____

ATTITUDE — Consider cooperation with manager and co-workers; receptiveness to suggestions and constructive criticism; attitude toward Practice; enthusiasm in attempts to improve performance.

❑ Needs much improvement   ❑ Needs improvement   ❑ Satisfactory
❑ Very good   ❑ Outstanding

Reason:____
____
____

TEAM EFFORT– LEADERSHIP — Consider ability to inspire teamwork, enthusiasm to work towards a common objective, desire to assume responsibility, ability to originate or develop ideas and get things started.

❑ Needs much improvement   ❑ Needs improvement   ❑ Satisfactory
❑ Very good   ❑ Outstanding

Reason:____
____
____

ADHERENCE TO POLICIES AND PROCEDURES — Consider adherence to practice personnel policies and procedures such as attendance, travel policies, and reporting deadlines.

❑ Needs much improvement   ❑ Needs improvement   ❑ Satisfactory
❑ Very good   ❑ Outstanding

Reason:____
____
____

Self-development activities of this employee (to be completed during interview).

____

____

____

____

PRESENT STATUS, NEEDS, AND PLAN OF ACTION

OVERALL EFFECTIVENESS — Considering the amount of experience on present job, check the rating which most nearly describes total current performance.

- ☐ Needs much improvement
- ☐ Needs improvement
- ☐ Satisfactory
- ☐ Very good
- ☐ Outstanding

What aspects of performance, if not improved, might hinder future development or cause difficulty in present classification (weakness of employee)?

____

____

____

____

____

What are greatest strengths of the employee?

____

____

____

____

____

Give specific plans you and your employee have made to improve work performance.

____

____

____

____

____

EMPLOYEE COMMENTS:

____

____

____

____

Forward completed performance appraisal to designated approval authority before reviewing with subject employee. After appraisal is approved, review contents of appraisal with subject employee and complete section concerning specific plans to improve performance. Have employee sign the form and then forward original appraisal to the personnel file. Retain a copy for your files.

Performance By Objective

OBJECTIVES FOR:

Use the spaces in the left column to list the most important Performance Management Objectives for the upcoming business year. Include specific business objectives and, as appropriate, one or two personal development objectives. After objectives are determined, the employee and manager should sign and retain a copy of the form. The right column will be used to summarize the employee's performance at year end.

OBJECTIVES	RESULTS/STATUS
1. _____________ Completion Date	
2. _____________ Completion Date	
3. _____________ Completion Date	
4. _____________ Completion Date	
5. _____________ Completion Date	
6. _____________ Completion Date	

EMPLOYEE COMMENTS:

EVALUATED BY:	TITLE:	DATE:
APPROVED:	TITLE:	DATE:
EMPLOYEE'S SIGNATURE (Does not necessarily indicate concurrence)	TITLE:	DATE:

SALARY CHANGE RECOMMENDATION

This request is not official until all approvals are indicated and a copy is returned to the manager/supervisor. Complete in duplicate and submit to Payroll Manager.

Date of Request: _____________________________   Date of Employment: _____________________________

Practice: ____

Employee: _________________________________   Department: _________________________________

LAST INCREASE, ANNUALIZED

FROM	TO	AMOUNT OF INCREASE	% INCREASE	DATE

PREVIOUS INCREASE, ANNUALIZED

FROM	TO	AMOUNT OF INCREASE	% INCREASE	DATE

RECOMMENDATION
SALARY ADJUSTMENT REQUEST - ANNUALIZED

FROM:	AMOUNT OF INCREASE:
TO:	PERCENT OF INCREASE: _______________ %

TITLE CHANGE: ☐ No   ☐ Yes / To:____

Comments:____

____

____

Signed: _________________________________   Approved: _________________________________
           Manager/Supervisor   Administrator

Effective Payroll Date: _____________________   Approved: _________________________________
                                                              Physician

CORRECTIVE ACTION FORM

Employee's Name: ____

Job Title: ____ Division: ________________

Hire Date: ____________________________

TYPE OF ACTION: (Check One)

☐ Verbal Warning   ☐ Final Warning   ☐ Discharge

☐ Written Warning   ☐ Disciplinary Suspension

PREVIOUS CORRECTION ACTIONS: (Type of Action, Offense, Date)

____

____

____

I. INCIDENT: Describe the situation (behavior, performance, policy violation, etc.) that occurred. Include date(s), time(s), locations(s), people involved, witnesses, effects of incident on employee's work or other employees, and all other relevant circumstances or contributing factors. Please be specific in stating observable behaviors and comments whenever possible.

____

____

____

____

____

____

____

____

____

II. GOALS AND TIME FRAME FOR IMPROVEMENT: What specific actions, within what time frame, are to be accomplished to improve the behavior/performance?

____

____

____

____

____

____

____

____

____

III. FOLLOW-UP REVIEW DATE: ___________________________

IV. CONSEQUENCES: What will happen if employee fails to meet the goals set within the designated time frames?

____
____
____
____
____
____
____
____
____

V. EMPLOYEE'S COMMENTS: My manager has reviewed the above situation with me and my comments are as follows:

____
____
____
____
____
____
____
____
____
____
____

Manager's Signature: ____ Date: __________________

I understand that my signature indicates only that this incident has been reviewed with me and does not indicate agreement or disagreement with the action taken.

Employee's Signature: ____ Date: __________________
(Not required for verbal warning)

TERMINATING EMPLOYEE CHECKLIST

Employee: _______________________________________

Date of Termination: _______________________________

ACTION	RESPONSIBILITY	✓
Keys Returned	Manager	
DOL State of Separation Notice	Manager	
Termination Date to Payroll Manager	Manager	
Termination Information (salary, vacation, etc.) to Payroll Manager	Manager	
Termination Letter		
Termination Memo to Staff	Manager	
Removal from Employee Roster		
Exit Interview Letter		
COBRA Form (for continuation of insurance)		
Exit Interview Letter Sent		
401(k) Plan		
Defined Benefit Plan		

PRACTICE MANAGEMENT STATISTICS

Category	National	My Office			
		1 Qtr.	2 Qtr.	3 Qtr.	4 Qtr.
Collections					
Total Annual Collections					
Refunds					
Net Collections					
Managed Care Collections (List each major plan separately)					
Expenses					
Total Expenses					
Total Overhead Percentages					
Salaries (%)					
Medical Supplies & Drugs (%)					
Administrative Supplies (%)					
Occupancy Expense (%)					
Malpractice Insurance (%)					
Legal & Accounting (%)					
Practice Statistics					
Staffing Ratio					
New patient visits/wk					
Established patient visits/wk					
Revenue per patient visit					
Cost per patient visit					
Average new patient charge					
Average established patient charge					
Collection Ratio					
Accounts Receivable Ratio					

MAJOR EXPENSES BY SPECIALTY

Expense Category	Cardiology	Family Medicine	GASTRO	Internal Medicine	OB/GYN	Opthal.	ENT	Pediatrics	Surgery General	Orthopedic
Personnel Salaries										
Personnel Benefits										
Rent										
Lab										
Medical Supplies										
Administrative Supplies										
Malpractice										
Legal and Accounting										
Promotions/Marketing										
Operating Overhead										

Used by Permission from Medical Group Management Association

PETTY CASH FUND

Date Starting: _______________________   Starting Amount: (A) _____________________________

Date Ending: _______________________   Ending Balance in Account: _____________________

DISBURSEMENTS LOG		
Date	**Reason**	**(A) Amount $**
Total Transactions: ________________		**Total (B):** $ ______________

Request for Petty Cash: Formula Starting Amount:

$ = (A)   ## (A) – (B) = (C)

Your Name: ____   Date: ____________________

SUMMARY REPORT FOR TRACKING PRACTICE GROWTH AND PROFITABILITY				
	GOAL	**CURRENT MONTH**	**PREV. MONTH**	**YTD**
BILLINGS				
COLLECTIONS				
COLLECTION PERCENTAGE (Fee-for-service cash collections ÷ Gross fee-for-service charges)				
TOTAL ACCOUNTS RECEIVABLE				
ACCOUNTS RECEIVABLE RATIO (Total Accounts Receivable ÷ Average monthly billings				
EXPENSE RATIO (Total office non-physician expense ÷ Total gross charges)				
PROFIT < LOSS > (Collections minus expenses)				
NET INCOME PERCENTAGE Total net income ÷ collections)				
NEW PATIENTS				
TOTAL PATIENT VISITS				

Patient Information Registration Form

Exhibit 5-1

PATIENT INFORMATION REGISTRATION FORM

(Please print clearly)

Patient's Full Name: _______________________________ Age: ______ DOB:_______________ Sex: ❑ M ❑ F

Address:_______________________________ City: _______________________ Zip: ___________

Home Phone: _______________________________ ❑ Married ❑ Single ❑ Divorced ❑ Separated ❑ Widowed

Social Security No.:_______________________________ Driver's License No.: _______________________

Patient's Employer: _______________________________ Phone No.:_______________________

Address:_______________________________ City: _______________________ Zip: ___________

Occupation: _______________________________

Spouse: _______________________________ Social Security No.: _______________________

Spouse's Employer: _______________________________ Phone: _______________________

Address:_______________________________ City: _______________________ Zip:___________

Occupation:_______________________________ Driver's License No.: _______________________

Family Physician: _______________________________ Referred By: _______________________

In case of emergency, contact (other than spouse): _______________________________

Address:_______________________________ City: _______________________ Zip: ___________

Relationship:_______________________________ Phone No.: _______________________

REFERRAL INFORMATION (Please tell us how you were referred to our practice)

Family Physician: _______________________________

Health Plan: _______________________________

Other Source: _______________________________

INSURANCE INFORMATION

Primary Coverage, Name of Carrier: Secondary Coverage, Name of Carrier:

_______________________________   _______________________________

Group No.: _______________________   Group No.: _______________________

Identification No.: _______________________   Identification No.: _______________________

Subscriber: _______________________   Subscriber: _______________________

Effective Date:_______________________   Effective Date:_______________________

Are you covered by Medicare? ❑ Yes ❑ No Medicare No: _______________________Railroad? _______________________

Are you covered by Medicaid? ❑ Yes ❑ No Please give secretary a current Medical Eligibility Form.

We ask all patients to show their insurance or managed care membership card so that we may make copies of them.

We cannot render services on the assumption that our charges will be paid by an insurance company. All services are charged directly to the patient, and he or she remains personally responsible for payment. As a courtesy, however, we will prepare any necessary reports and itemizations to assist in making collections from insurance companies and will credit any such collections to the patient's account.

PAYMENT AUTHORIZATION

I,_______________________ , hereby authorize_______________________ , M.D. to furnish information concerning my present illness. I direct the insurer to pay, without equivocation, directly to the physician, all benefits due him as a result of this claim. Although covered by insurance, I am aware that I am personally responsible for all charges. A photostatic copy of this authorization will be as valid as the original.

Signature of Patient: _______________________________ Date: _______________________

Guide to Estimate Times for Common Medical Office Procedures*

Procedure	Time in Minutes
Allergy Testing	30
Cast Change	30
Complete Physical Examination (CPX)	30 - 60
with Electrocardiogram (ECG)	+15
Dressing Change (with drain)	15
Hypertension Follow-up	10 - 15
Minor Surgery	30 - 60
Office Visit	
Brief	5 - 10
Intermediate (for acute illness)†	15 - 20
Extended	30+
Patient Teaching / Conference	30 - 60
Pelvic and Pap Test (P&P)	15 - 30
Prenatal Checkup	15 - 30
Replacement Suturing	30
Suture Removal	10 - 20

* The times given are approximate and may be adjusted to accommodate physician preference and patient needs.

† The intermediate visit is the most common. These breakdowns reflect standard manual recordkeeping categorizations.

Appointment Schedule **Exhibit 5-3**

APPOINTMENT SCHEDULE

Date: ___________________________

Time	Name	Chief Complaint	Home Phone	Work Phone

PATIENT SATISFACTION SURVEY

Below are a number of questions about your recent visit to our office. We want to provide the best service possible, but to do so we need to know what we are doing right and what needs improvement. Please take a few minutes to complete this survey and return it to us in the envelope provided. Your opinions are very important to us.

About yourself:

Age: ___________   Name (optional): ____ Sex: ______

Address: ____

Marital Status: ❑ Single   ❑ Married   ❑ Widow(er)

Name and Age of Spouse: ____

Names and Ages of Children: ____

Occupation: Yours: ______________________________ Spouse: __________________________________

Education: Yours:________________________________ Spouse: __________________________________

Best Times for Appointments: ____

Are we the main source of health care for your family?   ❑ Yes   ❑ No

If members of your family are seeing other physicians, please tell us who and why.

Spouse: ____

Children: ____

Other: ____

Type of Insurance:

❑ Blue Cross   ❑ HealthChoice   ❑ Aetna   ❑ Medicare   ❑ Medicaid   ❑ Self-pay   ❑ Other

About Our Physicians:

Which physician did you see?____

Please tell us how you would rate each of the following:

Scheduling	Excellent	Average	Poor
1. Promptness in which the phone was answered when you called the office			
2. Courtesy of the staff taking your call			
3. Efficiency of staff scheduling your appointment			
4. Availability of appointment times			
Physical Plant	**Excellent**	**Average**	**Poor**
5. Convenience of our location			
6. Ease of parking			
7. Cleanliness and comfort of the office			
8. Cleanliness of the restroom			
Front Office Personnel	**Excellent**	**Average**	**Poor**
9. Courtesy of the receptionist when you arrived at the office			
10. Courtesy and helpfulness of the business personnel			
11. Helpfulness of the staff in explaining your bill and payment responsibilities			
12. Accuracy of your bill			

Front Office Personnel (continued)	Excellent	Average	Poor
13. Helpfulness of the staff with insurance matters			
14. Ease of scheduling follow-up appointment time			
15. Ease of getting questions answered by phone about your bill			
16. Time you waited in the waiting room to see physician — how long? _______			
17. Time you waited in the examination room to see physician — how long?_______			
Doctors	Excellent	Average	Poor
18. Responsiveness and degree of caring the physician showed you			
19. Time spent with the physician? Length of time ____________			
20. Explanation by physician of your diagnosis			
21. How clearly did the physician answer your questions			
22. Explanation by physician of any follow-up visits			
23. Explanation by physician of any follow-up procedures			
24. Ability of the physician to communicate in layman s (e.g. understandable) terms			
25. Explanation by physician regarding medications			
26. Explanation by physician regarding test results			
27. Information provided by physician regarding preventive care			
Nurses	Excellent	Average	Poor
28. Attitude and expertise			
29. Respect for your sense of modesty and privacy			
30. Promptness of obtaining test results — who called with results? ____________			
31. Ease of getting questions answered by phone about follow-up procedures, medications or test results			
After-Hours and Weekend Care	Excellent	Average	Poor
32. Physician availability after hours			
33. Promptness and courtesy of answering service			
34. Speed with which physician returns your call			

Reason You Decided to Seek Medical Treatment in this Office.

❏ Near home or business ❏ Referral by another patient ❏ Referral by local medical society

❏ Yellow Pages listing ❏ Physician referral service ❏ Physician belongs to my insurance plan

❏ Referral by another physician; who?____

❏ Other ____

Do you have any other comments or suggestions to help us improve our service to you? ____________

____

____

____

____

____

PLEASE MAIL YOUR COMPLETED SURVEY IN THE POSTAGE PAID ENVELOPE PROVIDED. THANK YOU FOR TAKING THE TIME TO ANSWER THIS QUESTIONNAIRE. WE LOOK FORWARD TO SERVING YOU AGAIN.

HEALTH PLAN PROFILE

Plan Name: _________________________________ Telephone #: _____________________

Address: _________________________________

____

_________________________________ FAX #: _____________________

Provider Relations Representative:

____

Benefit Verification Number:____

Pre-certification/Authorization Telephone Number: _______________________________

AMOUNT

Plan Deductible: _______________________________________

Plan Copayment: _______________________________________

Hospital(s) within plan: _______________________________________

____

External Labs within plan: _______________________________________

External X-rays within plan: _______________________________________

Other Ancillary Facilities within plan: _______________________________________

Requirements   **YES**   **NO**

  Outpatient Authorization   _______   _______

  Inpatient Authorization   _______   _______

  Second Surgical Opinion   _______   _______

  Internal Lab   _______   _______

  Internal X-ray   _______   _______

Incident Report Form

Exhibit 7-1

INCIDENT REPORT FORM

Date of Complaint: _______________________________________ File/Medical Record No.: __________________

Patient's Name: ____

Address: ____

____

Telephone: ____

Person Taking Complaint: ____

Date Doctor Notified (should be same as above): Mo/Day/Yr: _____________________________________

Nature of Complaint (include dates, times, name of any person(s) involved): ________________________

____

____

____

____

____

Date of Response: ____

Response: ____

____

____

____

Follow-up Action/Date: ____

Resolution: ____

____

____

Signature of Person
Responding and Resolving: _______________________________________ Date: _______________________

PATIENT COMPLAINT LOG			
Patient Name	**Date**	**Date Doctor Notified**	**Person Taking Complaint**

(Via Certified Mail — Return Receipt Requested)

Date:

Dear ________________________ :
                patient's name

I find it necessary to inform you that I will no longer be able to provide medical care for you
because ________ *reason for discharge* ________ *(unless for reasons other than noncompliance)* ________ .

Since your condition requires continued medical attention, I suggest that you place yourself
under the care of another physician without delay. If you desire, I will be available for
emergency care and already scheduled appointments for a reasonable time after you receive this
letter, but in no event later than ________________ *(30 days from this date)* ________________ .

This should give you ample time to select a physician of your choice from the many competent
practitioners in this area. You may want to call the local county medical society at ____________
________ *phone number* ________ or ________ *the local hospital's* ________ physician referral service for
their assistance in locating a new physician. With your written authorization, I will make a copy
of your medical records available to your new physician.

Very truly yours,

____
                physician's name

(Source: Medical Association of Georgia Insurance Company)

To Dr. ____________________________ :

I authorize you to furnish a copy of the medical records of ____________________________

covering the period from __________________ , 19_____ to __________________ , 19_____

or to allow those records to be inspected or copied by __________________________ .

I release you from all legal responsibility or liability that may arise from this authorization.

Signed:____ Date:__________________

Witness:____

MEDICAL RECORDS CHECKLIST

	Yes	No	N/A
Patient name on all pages			
All pages secured with fasteners			
Forms organized with tabs for easy access			
Organized chronologically			
Legible entries			
Missed appointments documented			
Telephone message documented			
Allergies uniformly documented			
Entries dated, timed and initialed			
Dictation proofread and initialed			
Only standard abbreviations used			
Diagnostic reports initialed prior to filing			
Reason for visit documented			
Clinical findings (positive/negative) documented			
Treatment plan documented			
Entries are objective			
Patient instructions documented			
Patient education materials given/documented			
Medication List			
1. current			
2. prescriptions			
3. refills			
4. allergies			
Informed consent on chart			
Referral letters on chart			
Consultation reports on chart			
Problem list kept current			

MEDICATION RECORD

Patient Name: ____ Allergies: _____________________

Date of Birth: ____ Age: _________________________

Date	Medication	Dosage	Frequency	#	# Refills	Generic Y/N	Initial

Bibliography

Employee Termination Manual for Managers and Supervisors.
Chicago, IL: Commerce Clearing House, 1991.

Greenspan, Amy L. *Medical Employer's Guide.*
Bedford, TX: Summers Press, Inc., 1995.

Hubbartt, William S. *Performance Appraisal Manual for Managers and Supervisors.*
Chicago, IL: Commerce Clearing House, 1992.

Human Resources Management: Equal Employment Opportunity. Vol. II.
Chicago, IL: Commerce Clearing House, 1993.

Human Resources Management: Personnel Practices/Communications. Vols. I & II.
Chicago, IL: Commerce Clearing House, 1993.

Katz, Harvey P., M.D. *Telephone Medicine: Triage & Training — A Handbook for Primary Care Health Professionals.* F. A. Davis Co., 1990.

Sexual Harassment Manual for Managers and Supervisors.
Chicago, IL: Commerce Clearing House, 1991.

Woodke, Dale, R.N., N.P. *Medical Economics — Telephone Triage Protocols for Primary Care Centers.* July 10, 1995.

Workers' Compensation Manual for Managers and Supervisors.
Chicago, IL: Commerce Clearing House, 1992.

Resources

Stanton L. Burnette, CIC, Burnette Insurance, 1938 Old Norcross Road,
Lawrenceville, Georgia 30244

Index

A

Accident/Injury Report 22, 103-105

Accounting Fees..64

Accounts Payable..3, 66-67

Accounts Receivable...................................3-4, 68-72

ADA 19, 25-26

ADEA 19, 26-27

Administrative Employee 30

Advertisements to Hire Employees......................27, 35

Age Discrimination in Employment Act 19, 26-29

Age Discrimination 35, 38

Americans with Disabilities Act of 1990.....19, 25-26, 29

Applicants...35-36, 38-39

Applications for Employment...................................27

Appointment Scheduling and
Registration Policy.......................................74-76, 129

Appraisal..34, 45-49, 115

At-Will Contracts..31

Attendance Records..27

Authorization for Release of Medical Records...........136

B

Bartering 63

Benchmarking..57-58

Benefits 55

Billing and Collections....................................61-62, 92

Bloodborne Pathogens Standard 23, 28, 74, 106-110

Budget...57

C

Candidate Profile 34-35

Certificates of Age 27

Child Labor..28-29

Civil Rights Act 19

COBRA 23

Collecting 70

Communication 9-12, 34

Confidentiality 94

Consent to Treatment..95-96

Consolidated Omnibus Budget
Reconciliation Act of 1985 19

Corrective Action Form 120

Credentialing of Health Care Providers 41

Curriculum Vitae...44

D

Demotions 27

Disability Discrimination 29, 38, 78

Disciplinary Action...51-52

Discrimination Complaint Records and Actions..........27

Dual Capacity Doctrine 21, 23

E

EEOC...19, 29

Emergencies...93

Employee Conduct 55

Employee Handbook..53-55

Employee Leasing 42

Employee Performance Appraisal Form 115

Employee Safety Orientation Checklist................21, 102

Employment Categories.......................................30-31

Employment Contracts 27

Employment History..27

Environment...93

EOBs 40

Equal Employment 29

Equal Employment Opportunity Act of 1972 19

Equal Pay Act...19, 28

Equity Theory 8

ERISA Plan Disclosures..27

Executive Employee..31

Exempt 30

Explanation of Benefits...40

Exposure Incident 23

    Protocol...106

    Report...107

F, G

Facility Evaluation 80
Facility Management 76-77
Fair Debt Collection Act 92
Fair Labor Standards Act 17-18, 27-28
Family Medical Leave Act of 1993 20
Fees 71-72
Fixed Expenses 65
FLSA 17-18
Form I-9 27
Guide to Estimated Times for
Common Medical Procedures 128

H, I, J, K

Handling Patient Complaints 94
HIV/AIDS 97
Health Plan Profile 87, 132
Hiring 27, 33-42
Immigration Documentation 27
Immigration Reform and Control Act 27
Incident Report Form 133
Independent Contractors 42
Informed Consent to Treat 95-96, 98, 109
Injury Summary 28
Insurance
      Malpractice...88
      Professional Liability....................................88
      Workers' Compensation 20-23
Interior Office Checklist 79-84
Interviewing 3, 4-5, 36-38
Inventory Control 62-63
Job Description 2, 33-34, 111-114
Job Offer 39, 43

L, M

Layoffs 27
Leadership...5-6
Legal Fees..64
Letter of Employment 39, 43
Major Expenses by Specialty....................60, 124
Malpractice 88
Managing Conflict..7
Marketing in Managed Care Market 86-87
Maslow's Hierarchy of Needs.................................8-9
Medical Professional Liability..................................64

Medical Equipment

Medical Equipment 93
Medical Record(s) 2, 28, 97, 137-138
Minimum Wage...17
Misconduct Problems..51

N, O

Nonexempt...30-31
Occupancy Expense..63
Occupational Safety & Health Administration...23, 28, 74
Office Environment 76
Operating Budget 57
Order Point System...63
Order, Shipping, Billing, and Payment Records...........28
Ordering Logs 63
OSHA 23, 73, 74
Outsourcing...42, 61
Overtime...17-18

P, Q

Patient Billing...69, 92
Patient Complaint Log 134
Patient Cost Analysis...66
Patient Information 69, 127
Patient Satisfaction Survey 81, 130
Patient Services and Amenities................................84
Patient's Obligations...96
Patient's Rights 95
Patient's Release of Information.............................97-98
Pay Determination...34
Pay Rate 27
Payroll..2, 3, 62, 67
Payroll Records..28
Performance Appraisal 34, 45-49
Performance Problems 51
Personnel Costs 59-60
Personnel File 40
Petty Cash 64, 125
Physical Examination Results...................................28
Physical Plant 77
Physician's Obligations..96
Policies and Procedures Manual 73
Polygraph Testing...29
Post-Exposure Incident
      Exposed Employee Incident Form 110
      Source Individual Incident Form.......................109
Practice Management Statistics Form 123

Precertification 87
Pregnancy Discrimination Act of 1978 19
Probationary Period 40-41
Procedure Manual 73
Procedure Unit Cost 72
Professional Employee 30
Promotions 27
Purchasing 61

R

Reasonable Accommodation 25-26, 78
Reception 76
Recruiting 34
References 39
Registration 76
Resumés 35
Revenues 65
Rights of the Patient 95

S

Safety 20, 55
Salary Administration 45-50
Salary Change Recommendation 119
Sale and Purchase Agreements 28
Sample Discharge Letter 135
Scheduling 74-76, 91
Service Contracts 64
Sexual Harassment 24-25
Staff Meetings 8-9
Staffing Ratios by Specialty 59-60
Summary Report for Tracking Practice
Growth and Profitability 126

T–Z

Team Building..7
Telephone Screening 36
Telephone Triage Guidelines 88-89
Terminating Employee Checklist 122
Terminating the Physician/Patient
Relationship 70, 94-95
Termination 27, 52
Tests 28
Time Management 12-16
Title VII 24, 27-28

Training 27-28, 34, 44-45
Transfers 27
U.S. Department of Labor 29
Variable Expenses 65
Vendor Relations 62
Vietnam Era Veteran's Readjustment Assistance Act ...27
Wage-Hour Law Compliance 28, 34
Wage Records 28
Walk-ins 74-75
Workers' Compensation 20-23
Written Collection Policy 69
Written Financial Payment Policy 69